deutsche
forschungsgemeinschaft

conference on population monitoring methods for detecting increased mutation rates

JAHRESKONFERENZ 1975

zentrallaboratorium
für mutagenitätsprüfung

CIP-Kurztitelaufnahme der Deutschen Bibliothek

Conference on Population Monitoring Methods for Detecting Increased Mutation Rates ⟨1975, Freiburg, Breisgau⟩
Conference on Population Monitoring Methods for Detecting Increased Mutation Rates: Jahreskonferenz 1975, Zentrallaboratorium für Mutagenitätsprüfung Freiburg / Dt. Forschungsgemeinschaft. – Bonn-Bad Godesberg: Deutsche Forschungsgemeinschaft; Boppard: Boldt, 1977.
(Mitteilung / Kommission für Mutagenitätsfragen; 4)
ISBN 3-7646-1693-8

NE: Zentrallaboratorium für Mutagenitätsprüfung ⟨Freiburg, Bresgau⟩; Deutsche Forschungsgemeinschaft

Harald Boldt Verlag
5407 Boppard, Postfach 110
ISBN: 3 7646 1693 8

53 Bonn-Bad Godesberg 1, Kennedyallee 40
Telefon (0 22 21) 871
Telegrammanschrift: Forschungsgemeinschaft
Herstellung: boldt druck boppard gmbh

CONTENTS

FOREWORD

The "Zentrallaboratorium für Mutagenitätsprüfung" (ZLM) has established the tradition of organizing biannual work-shops on fundamental questions of mutagenesis. Thus, a conference on "Human Population Monitoring" was held in Freiburg from May 26th to 31st, 1975. The collaborators of the ZLM wish to express their indeptedness to Mrs. Dr. Lili Schoeller, for the scientific and technical organization of this meeting.

Through this publication the ZLM would like to make the main aspects of this meeting available to a larger public.

PROGRAM

Conference on Human Population Monitoring
Methods for Detecting Increased Mutation Rates
(May 26–31, 1975)

I. INTRODUCTORY SURVEY

What can we predict about the impact on populations of an increased mutation rate?

H. B. Newcombe	"Priorities in assessing the impact on human populations of an increased mutation rate"
J. V. Neel	"The monitoring of human populations for mutations affecting protein structure and/or functions: problems and prospects"
S. Abrahamson	"Risk estimates for man from chemical-environmental mutagens"

II. CHROMOSOME AND GENE MUTATIONS IN POPULATION SAMPLES

H. J. Evans	"Chromosomal and DNA damage in peripheral blood lymphocytes of individuals exposed to known or suspected mutagens: Problems and perspectives"
A. Schinzel and W. Schmid	"An evaluation of the blood culture method: Cytogenetic findings in lymphocyte cultures of 61 patients treated with cytostatic drugs"
W. Schmid	"Prenatal chromosome analysis. Data from our own laboratory and review"
H. Galjaard	"Possibilities and limitations in prenatal diagnosis: A survey of about 400 cases"
W. Tünte	"Paternal age as a possible means for detecting spontaneous mutations"

III. IMMUNE REACTION SYSTEMS

A. Lengeróva	"Advantages and disadvantages of histocompatibility systems in monitoring increased mutation rates"

K. Bender	"Heterozygosity at the HL-A gene loci in children and old people"
E. Albert	"Closely linked genes in the major histocompatibility complex in man"
E. Günther	"Genetic complementation of IR-genes" (short introduction)

IV. ELECTROPHORETIC SYSTEMS

K. Altland	"Screening for new mutations at the protein level. Large number versus small number of loci to be tested: A problem of economy"
J. Klose	"Testing for point mutations by protein mapping"
H. Galjaard	"Studies on genetic heterogeneity in inborn errors of metabolism using somatic cell hybridization"
C. H. Langley	"Projected advantages and disadvantages in possible somatic cell mutation monitoring"
V. Neuhoff	"Microelectrophoresis for rapid fractionation of RNA, proteins, enzymes and isoenzymes"

V. HEREDITARY CLINICAL SYNDROMS

K.-H. Degenhardt	"Diagnosis of hereditary clinical syndroms with special regard to slight deviations"
W. Engel	"A new type of genetically determined diseases: Hormone receptor defects"

VI. ORGANIZATION OF MONITORING PROGRAMS

K.-H. Degenhardt	"Etiology of congenital anomalies in a cohort of prospective pregnancies and their outcomes"

VII. EVALUATION OF THE DATA.
CONSTRUCTION OF FEASIBLE MODELS

J. F. Crow	(summing up)

Organization L. Schoeller

(Acknowledgement is due to our secretary, Miss Renate Altmann, for her very competent and kind assistance.)

INTRODUCTION

Following the recommendation of the Senate Commission for Mutagenicity Problems of the Deutsche Forschungsgemeinschaft, conferences on related topics are held periodically in the Zentrallaboratorium für Mutagenitätsprüfung (ZLM). These international conferences aim at exchanging information on basic research and methodology in the field of mutagenicity. Emphasis is given to free discussion; thus, apart from the more general introductory presentations at the beginning of the conference, all contributions dealing with specific subjects are meant to induce extensive discussion.

SPECIAL PURPOSE OF THIS CONFERENCE

The main object of the conference in 1975 was to collect detailed information on currently available methodology for detecting increased mutation rates, to critically discuss each method's advantages and disadvantages, and to find out whether the participants would agree on the feasibility and the importance of a human population monitoring program. The question whether or not there is a detectable mutation increase in the human population induced by environmental agents is a fundamental one for the ZLM, since the purpose in establishing and maintaining this institute has been based on it's contribution in protecting the human population against mutations induced by chemicals from our environment. The many difficulties, scientifical, methodical and political, involved in this task are well known.

In his contribution "General Remarks and Conclusions" the Chairman of the conference, Dr. J. F. Crow, assesses: "What we most need to know is the relationship between mutation rate and human impairment. Rather than to classify diseases and other deleterious traits as to whether they are genetic or not, what we need to do is classify them as to the extent that they are maintained by recurrent mutation. In other words, how can we estimate the proportion of human genetic impairment that would increase linearly with the mutation rate? Such research will not be easy."

GENERAL REMARKS AND CONCLUSIONS

JAMES F. CROW

It is not my purpose to give a general summary of what has been said at this conference; the individual papers speak for themselves and attest to the wide variety of subjects dealt with. Rather, I shall try to assess what seem to me to be the general conclusions regarding population monitoring that have grown out of the discussions.

Let me emphasize at the outset that detecting a mutation rate increase by population monitoring is not the way of choice. If a mutagen is discovered in this way, damage has already been done. It is far better to discover mutagenic properties of chemicals before they come into widespread use; then the appropriate decision can be made in advance. It is quite proper that most of the emphasis has thus far been placed on inexpensive, efficient and relevant tests for mutagenicity, using systems based on experimental organisms and laboratory tests.

In 1966 the Genetics Study Section of the United States National Institutes of Health, following a conference held at the Jackson Laboratory in Maine, made four recommendations [1]: The first was that a register of mutagenic chemicals be kept and the information made generally available. The second was that mutagenicity testing be made a routine part of the testing of chemicals used in foods and drugs, or to which large numbers of persons may be exposed for other reasons. The third was that research to develop more sensitive and cheaper assays of mutagenicity and chromosome breakage, or assays based on organisms more closely related to man, be encouraged and supported. The fourth recommendation was that the feasibility of genetic monitoring of the human population be explored.

It is gratifying that the first three of these recommendations have been put into effect on a wide scale and with a high level of international cooperation. It is also gratifying that many new chemicals are being tested and that many old ones, conventionally regarded as safe, are being reappraised. There have been many impressive technical improvements. Although progress may not have been as rapid as some would hope, the program is clearly off and running in many parts of the world.

The fourth recommendation is the basis of this conference. Despite a scientifically advanced, extensive, and conscientious program for detecting mutagens in advance of their use, there is always the possibility that a potent mutagen will evade discovery and that large numbers of persons will be exposed. So we need to give serious thought to ways of detecting an increased mutation rate and, should this be found, of identifying the cause.

ATTRIBUTES OF A GOOD MONITORING SYSTEM

I have previously discussed the attributes of a desirable test system [2] and others have presented similar ideas. Some important criteria are:

1. *The system should be relevant.* What we fear for future generations is disease, pain, reduced life expectancy and other major and minor impediments to human fulfillment. We don't know the relative contribution of dominant, X-linked and autosomal recessive, and polygenic mutants to the mutational load; nor do we know how to assess the relative importance of cytogenetic changes, although some cytogenetic statistics are now quite solid. Since we cannot measure damage to future generations in a tangible way, the most relevant thing to do is to monitor the genetic changes themselves. If the monitoring system does not measure the mutation rate itself, it should measure something very higly correlated with it.

2. *The system should give results promptly.* The more rapidly the system can sense a mutation rate increase, the better. This implies that detection of germinal mutations should emphasize tests on newborns and young children, or embryos.

3. *The system should be sensitive.* It should be able to detect a small change in the current mutation rate. Any system for detecting germinal mutations is limited by the population available. Somatic systems, on the other hand, sacrifice relevance.

4. *The system should detect a wide spectrum of genetic changes.* This means that it must detect cytogenetic changes, deletions, frame shifts, base changes – as many kinds of genetic changes as possible. More than one system will probably be needed to meet the various expected contingencies, for we can expect different environmental chemicals to act in different ways.

5. *The system should maximize the chance of detecting the cause of*

a mutation rate increase. Simply detecting an increase in the mutation rate is not enough, for we should like to eliminate the cause. A clue is likely to come from geographical localization, identification with users of some food or drug, association with some profession or some industry, or perhaps association with some cultural or economic group. This is difficult to plan for, but it is clear that only quite sensitive systems could detect a change of mutation rate in a small group. One of the great advantages of international cooperation in mutation testing is that a change in one country and not in others may enhance the chance of finding the cause.

6. *The system should be available now, or in the near future.* It may be necessary to go ahead with rather poor systems and modify or replace them, rather than wait for future basic discoveries to yield much better techniques. Although better methods are sure to come, the problem does not permit a leisurely wait. It is *most* important that any monitoring systems not be frozen by custom or regulation so that changes are difficult.

These 6 criteria seem to me to be the most important, but there are others that also deserve some consideration.

7. *The system should be simple to use.* If it is simple and foolproof, if it can be carried by non-professional personnel, if it can be automated and rely on instrumentation, it will be more reliable and easier to put into effect – to say nothing of saving costs.

8. *The cost should be reasonable.* Although the problem is important enough to warrant substantial expenditures, there is clearly a limit, both of money and trained manpower.

9. *Other things being comparable, a system with other benefits is preferred.* For example, monitoring newborns for physical abnormalities might not be worth the expense solely as a mutation-monitoring system, but if this were combined with a system for detecting teratogens it might be feasible. The high correlation between mutagenicity and carcinogenicity suggests that a mutation-detecting system might do double duty by detecting carcinogens, and *vice versa.* Similarly, a system that would yield other data of basic or practical interest is to be preferred. For example, a system designed to monitor the mutation rate by using biochemical markers might be partially justified by the information it could give regarding the normal mutation rate and by the discovery of new kinds of mutations of basic or medical importance.

HOW WELL DO EXISTING METHODS MEET THESE CRITERIA?

The systems that have been discussed at this conference, and which seem most ready to be put to use, can be classified in a 2 x 2 table.

	A Cytogenetic	B Genetic
I. Transmitted	Cytogenetic monitoring of newborn	1. Sentinel phenotypes 2. Biochemical mutants
II. Not transmitted	Cytogenetic monitoring of somatic cells	Somatic mutation studies

There is also a C category: Indirect methods, about which I shall say a few words later.

Let me now discuss each of the four compartments in the Table.

IA. *Cytogenetic monitoring of newborn.* It is clear from Dr. Evans' discussion that this is technically feasible. It meets very well the criteria of (1) relevance, (2) promptness, and (6) immediate availability. It does not detect a wide spectrum of changes, but it is not designed to do so. It detects its part of the spectrum of genetic damage directly and accurately. The system is somewhat insensitive, since it must depend on the individual infant as the unit; so numbers become a limiting factor. It is also expensive. It is available now and techniques steadily improve.

IIA. *Cytogenetic monitoring of somatic cells.* This is good from the standpoint of (2) promptness, (3) sensitivity, (5) opportunity to find the cause, and (6) availability. It is much more sensitive than monitoring for germinal changes, since the cell is the unit rather than the person. It is important to establish the extent of the correlation of germinal and somatic mutation rates. There are real difficulties caused by the large variance in number of mutants in clonally multiplying cells, but this can be met in several ways. One of the best would be successive measurements on the same persons. This would offer the best chance of identifying the time of a mutation rate increase and identifying the cause. As Dr. Evans has emphasized, interchanges seem excellent and sister-strand exchange promising from the standpoint of sensitivity and low background noise.

IB. *Monitoring for transmitted genetic changes.* There have been two systems advocated. The first is *Sentinel Phenotypes.* This is good from the standpoint of (1) relevance and (6) availability of techniques. But it is poor from almost every other standpoint. It could be fairly prompt if newborns provided most of the information; even so, it could be measuring mutation rate increases in the parents decades before. There is a paucity of phenotypes that meet stringent criteria for dominant inheritance, high penetrance, ability to rule out errors in paternity, and ease of diagnosis. The system would be expensive if it were done a scale large enough to be at all sensitive. Finally, it offers little or no chance of detecting the cause. The concensus of this meeting seems to be that the system would have to have at least partial justification for other reasons to merit its being put into effect. It might be made part of a teratogen detection system, or an epidemiological survey.
The use of *Biochemical Mutation Monitoring* has been extensively discussed. This conference has brought out some methods for technical improvement and lowering of costs. It has also pointed out possibilities for increasing the number of loci monitored. The spectrum of effects may not be as wide as might be desired, for only mutants producing structural changes in the protein molecule are likely to be detected. So far the system would be very expensive, insensitive, and would offer very little chance of detecting the cause. On the other hand, as Dr. Neel has argued, one can count on steady technical improvements, decreased costs, and increasing effectiveness as more and more loci are included. For one thing the troublesome problem of mistaken parentage can be reduced to an acceptable minimum with a large enough number of factors. And, as I mentioned earlier, if such a program were put into effect it would yield by-products in the form of information about normal mutation rates and new kinds of genetic variants.

IIB. *Monitoring for somatic mutation.* This was not discussed extensively at the conference, but it seems to me to be the most promising in the long run. The thymidine kinase and guanine-hypothxanthine phosphoribosyl transferase (HGPRT) systems, and others certain to be developed in the near future, offer chances for sensitive tests for somatic mutations, The most obvious way to get more information from each person is to use somatic cells. Of course, there are difficulties. One is the kind of statistical problem that arises in any study of mutants in a growing population of cells. There is also the question of relevance. A most urgent necessity is the correlation of somatic and germinal mutation rates to see if the responses to mutagens are parallel; such studies could be done with mice. Assuming that such a correlation exists, this should be a very valuable adjunct to germinal systems. In my opinion this is the most promising direction for research. Only somatic systems offer any real hope of detecting local increases in mutation rates and finding the causes.

INDIRECT METHODS

This was not much discussed at the conference, but I think it deserves mention nevertheless. One possibility that has been mentioned several times in the past few years and applied in some cases is the search for mutagens in human tissues. It is a simple task to determine if human blood or urine contains substances that are mutagenic in sensitive microbial test systems. This is analogous to the host-mediated assay.

Needless to say, there is much uncertainty as to whether compounds that are eaten or inhaled, or which otherwise get into the body, are mutagenic originally and converted into something harmless or were originally harmless and converted into mutagens. We are interested, of course, in those compounds that are mutagenic in the body, however they got to be that way. It is quite likely that differences between humans and test systems based on simpler organisms (particularly eukaryotes, such as yeast or Neurospora) lie more in the intermediate metabolism of ingested compounds than in their effect on the DNA. I think that monitoring human fluids is a very feasible operation. It is untested as to relevance, but it has all the other positive qualities that I mentioned before.

SOME GENERAL REMARKS

What we fear cannot be measured directly. Our concern is that an increased mutation rate will cause premature death, disease, and other burdens in future generations. But these are likely to be so diluted in space and time and so thoroughly interspersed with similar conditions from other causes that even a substantial mutation rate increase could go undetected for several generations.

Dr. Newcombe has called our attention to the shaky empirical base for any quantitative estimates of human mutational damage, even that which occurs naturally. The most tangible and most immediate effect would be that from severe dominant diseases. But the recent Canadian studies that Newcombe mentions suggest that this component may be a substantially smaller part of human disease than the earlier studies from Northern Ireland had indicated. X-linked recessives are somewhat comparable to autosomal dominants in that their incidence and time of expression are somewhat predictable from knowledge of mutation rates. They also have much more similar frequencies in the two studies. Aneuploidy syndromes also can be directly measured and their harm assessed. Autosomal recessives are expressed on the average so far in the future as to make us quite uncertain as to the extent to which they should be taken into account; certainly they deserve less emphasis than dominants whose expression is much sooner. The most difficult aspect of mutation to assess is the cumulative impact of many individually mild mutants. We know that in Drosophila such mutations are very frequent. Yet, as Newcombe has emphasized, mouse experiments designed to measure such effects have failed to find them even in mice exposed for many generations to heavy doses of radiation.

What we most need to know is the relationskhip between mutation rate and human impairment. Rather than to classify diseases and other deleterious traits as to whether they are genetic nor not, what we need to do is classify them as to the extent that they are maintained by recurrent mutation. In other words, how can we estimate the proportion of human genetic impairment that would increase linearly with the mutation rate? Such research will not be easy. We don't even have a solid basis of normal incidence of genetic disease, as Newcombe has so effectively pointed out.

There is, therefore, much room for uncertainty and disagreement about the magnitude of the mutation problem. But, there seems to be little disagreement as to the direction of the effect. We all believe that any increase in the mutation rate is undesirable, although we are not sure *how* undesirable.

My own view for several years has been that the ideal human mutation rate for the present and the foreseeable future is zero. There is already more genetic variability in the population than is needed for any reasonable contingency that we can anticipate. If the mutation rate were to drop to zero, the only way we would notice this would be by the decrease in frequency of some of our worst diseases. A corollary of this view is that the discovery of a safe antimutagen could be of great human benefit.

In the absence of any ability to control the spontaneous rate the most we can do is keep the rate from becoming higher. This requires some kind of policy that is generally agreed upon. We have such a policy for radiation. It may not be ideal, but we can at least be assured that if current radiation protection standards in effect in many parts of the world are adhered to, man-made radiation dosage will remain less than that from background radiation. The mutations thus induced are no greater than the number that we have experienced from background radiation over many generations. This is thought to be a small fraction of the mutations due to causes other than radiation. The radiation protection standards provide a level of mutation that a society can reasonably accept in return for the benefits of radiation; but this does not, of course, mean that we should relax our efforts to make the exposure still less.

With chemical mutagens we are on much less solid ground, for we don't have anything comparable to background radiation to use as a standard. Perhaps, as has been independently suggested by several people (see, for example, [3]), the permissible level of chemical mutagens can be somehow linked to radiation protection standards. By defining chemical mutation damage in terms of equivalently effective radiation doses, we can bring both causes into simultaneous view and set an overall standard that includes both. The units of measurement for chemicals could be some form of radion-equivalent and the acceptable dose could be related to background radiation.

I do not to imply that the problems of definition would be simple, for we certainly shall find non-comparability between radiation and chemical effects in different systems and at different concentrations. If the difficulties are so great as to make the system unfeasible, then perhaps we can try to use the human spontaneous mutation rate as a standard, trying always to keep the induced rate substantially lower than this.

FINAL REMARK

I emphasized earlier that one desirable attribute of a monitoring system, particularly during its developmental stages, is that it has beneficial side effects, such as contributions to fundamental knowledge. A similar principle is abundantly illustrated by this conference. Many of the subjects discussed are ancillary to the direct question of mutation monitoring. Yet, some of them may well lay the foundation for future monitoring techniques. The finding of more kinds of genes that might some time be built into test systems enhances the efficiency and the width of the spectrum of effects measured. New techniques offer possibilities for making the tests more efficient and for new, innovative directions. A conference such as this should not be judged solely by its contributions to the immediate problem; in the long run some of the findings that I have omitted may turn out to be the most important.

REFERENCES

[1] Crow, J. F.: Chemical risk to future generations. Scientist and Citizen 10, 113–117. 1968.

[2] Crow, J. F.: Human population monitoring. In Chemical Mutagens, Edited by A. Hollaender. Plenum Press, N. Y. Pp. 591–605. 1971.

[3] Environmental mutagenic hazards. Report of Committee 17 of the Environmental Mutagen Society, J. W. Drake, chairman. Science 187, 503–514. 1975.

QUADRATIC ANALYSIS OF THE INDUCTION OF SPECIFIC LOCUS MUTATIONS IN THE MOUSE

S. ABRAHAMSON, P. OFTEDAL, K. SANKANARAYAN, and S. WOLFF
(Communicated by James F. Crow)

The genetic effects of ionizing radiation in mice have been studied under many different experimental conditions [4, 7, 8, 11, see 14 for review]. Most of the data, which deal with mutation yields obtained with a specific locus test in the mouse [6], form a major element in the evaluation of possible genetic effects of radiation in humans [2, 4]. The mutagenic efficiency of radiation has varied with the experimental conditions, and no unifying interpretation for the data has been available. The mutations have commonly been considered to be one-hit events, and to account for protraction and fractionation effects, sensitivity differences between sexes, etc., various mechanisms such as differential intracellular repair [10] cell stage variation [7] cell selection [1] and cell synchronization [8] have been invoked. An alternative explanation has been offered [13, 15] based on X-ray-induced specific locus mutations being mainly two-hit deletions.

We have examined the data from Tables 13, 14, and 16 of UNSCEAR [14] as well as more recently published data [3, 4] and now find* that if the mutation yield versus dose is expressed as a simple quadratic

$$Y = C + \alpha D + \beta D^2$$

it is possible to make quantitative estimates of the yields of mutations obtained under different regimes of irradiation. In the equation Y = the expected yield of mutations, C = control rate, D = the dose of sparsely ionizing radiation, and α and β are the coefficients of induction. This expression is consistent with the interpretation that the mutations are largely one-hit [5] and two-hit [15] deletions.

---

* Much of this analysis was carried out during a meeting of a Genetics Task Group of Committee I of the International Commission on Radiological Protection (ICRP).

The work of SA and SW was supported by the United States Energy Research and Development Administration.

Because the data which are represented in Table I have been obtained under a variety of conditions, and there are such large statistical errors associated with the points, they can be interpreted in many ways. In the female, however, the use of the quadratic model for mutation induction provides a reasonable approximation for most of the data. Three items (items 6, 7, and 8) contain fewer mutations than predicted by the formula. These data come from very low dose rate experiments in which the total time taken to administer the radiation meant that the sampled oocytes included cells irradiated in the apparently insensitive stage [1, 10]. In the male, the use of the quadratic model does not provide as close an approximation as it does in the female. This is particularly noticeable after acute exposures of about 600 R or exposures of 1000 R either unfractionated (item 16a) or fractionated into two 500 R exposures with only a two hour interval (16b). Under the latter conditions the dose effect curve is distorted and the yields of mutations are even lower than after 600 R [9]. This factor, which has been attributed to cell killing [7], contributes to the lessened precision of the estimates for the male.

The values for α and β used in the estimation of the expected results are presented in Table II. For the female data the estimation of α and β was determined from items 1 and 2 of Table I by a least squares regression analysis of all four points. The data were derived from irradiation of maturing oocytes. In males the α term was taken directly from Searle [12] and the β term was calculated from the data observed at 300 R (item 11) which is the lowest acute dose used and the point at which the effects of cell killing would be minimized.

The values for α and β that are presented in Table II have proven useful in making risk estimates on the genetic effects of radiation. The α term can form the basis for estimating the doubling dose for sparsely ionizing radiation under low dose and low dose rate conditions, as well as the RBE for densely ionizing radiations.

Table 1

Item	Sex	Experimental Conditions	Mutants/ Total	Mutation Per Locus: Induced[a] rate x 10^{-5}	Expected rate x 10^{-5}	Ratio Exp/In	Reference
1	♀[b]	Control[c]	1/164993[d]	0.086			14
2	♀	50R x-ray at 90R/min	13/180472[d]	0.94	1.30	1.4	14
	♀	200 R x-ray at 90R/min	21/37297[d]	7.96	7.90	0.99	14
	♀	400R x-ray at 90R/min	23/14842[d]	22.1	22.2	1.0	14
3	♀	400R x-ray at 90R/min 8x50R, 75 minute intervals	19/27906	9.6	11.4	1.2	14
4	♀	400R x-ray at 90R/min 2x200R, 24 hour interval	9/6086	21.0	16.0	0.76	14
5	♀	400R γ-rays, .8R min 8.3 hours exposure	7/20827	4.7	9.8[f]	2.1	14
6	♀	600R γ-rays, .05R/min 12 days - 16 hr exposure	1/10117	1.3	14.7[g]	11.0	14
7	♀	258R γ-rays, .009R/min > 20 days exposure	1/8373	1.62	6.32[g]	3.9	14
8	♀	400R γ-rays, .009R/min > 31 days exposure	1/15195	0.85	9.8[g]	12.0	14
9	♂	Control (Oak Ridge & Harwell)	39/688921	0.81	0.0	–	14
10	♂	Dose range 37.5R-861R, γ-rays Dose rates .001-.009R/min 25-429 days			$\alpha = .0066$[h]	–	12
11	♂	300R, x-ray at 80–1000R/min[i]	64/103755[j]	8.0	8.0	–	14

12	♂	600R, x-ray 90R/min	111/119326	12.5	28.4	2.2[k]	14
12a	♂	670, x-ray 60–70R/min	12/11138	14.6	34.5	2.4[k]	4, 12
12b	♂	636R, γ-ray 17R/min	11/12021	12.3	31.3	2.5[k]	4
13	♂	600R, x-ray 80-90R/min 100+500, 24 hr. interval	42/24811	23.4	21.4	.91	14
14a	♂	624R, γ-ray, 60 daily doses 10.4 Rad at 17R/min 5 consecutive days each wk.	7/23982	3.4	4.55	1.3	4
14b	♂	600R, γ-ray, 90 daily doses at .008R/min=6.67 Rad/day	5/22682	2.3	3.96	1.7	4
14c	♂	600R, γ-ray, .05-.07 Rad/min 50R/day, once each wk X 12 wk	10/22816	5.5	3.96	.72	4
15	♂	600R, x-ray, 50R at 60R/min once ea. wk. x 12 wks.	16/18,119	11.8	5.97	.5	14
16a	♂	1000R, x-ray 80-90R/min	29/44649	8.47	73.6	8[k]	14
16b	♂	1000R, x-ray 80-90R/min 2x500R 2 hr interval	12/14879	10.7	73.6	7[k]	14
17a	♂	1000R, x-ray 80-90R/min 2x500R, 24 hr interval[l]	55/16626	46.5	40.	.86	3
17b	♂	1000R, x-ray, 76R/min 2x500R, 4 day interval	11/7168	21.1	40.	1.9	3
17c	♂	1000R, x-ray, 76R/min 2x500R, 7 day interval	11/8271	18.2	40.	2.2	3
17d	♂	1000R, x-ray, 90R/min 600 + 400 > 15 wk interval	10/4904	28.3	41.4	1.5	14
18a	♂	1000R, x-ray, 80-90R/min 5x200R, 24 hr interval	16/8588	25.8	20.0	.78	14
18b	♂	1000R, x-ray, 80-90R/min .5x200R weekly interval	15/10968	18.7	20.0	1.1	14

FOOTNOTES TO TABLE 1

a Corrected for control value.

b Analysis is restricted to litters conceived within seven weeks of irradiation period; litters conceived after 7 weeks sample oocytes in dictyate (immature stage) of apparently very low mutability.

c Restricting the control value to the cell population at risk (i. e. non-proliferating oocytes), and therefore eliminating a cluster of six identical mutants of oogonial or pre-oogonial origin.

d These experimental results are used to calculate the α and β terms for maturing oocytes.

e Assuming α and β term for each fraction, and additivity between fractions.

f Assuming no interaction, and therefore using only the α term.

g For exposures lasting several weeks or longer, analysis becomes difficult due to a mixture of oocytes irradiated in the dictyate stage, which is of extremely low apparent mutability [Para. 173, in ref. 14].

h Calculated from the linear regression on ten different experimental values in Searle [12], confidence values not given.

i Pooled data from two Russell experiments.

j This experimental result is used for calculating the β term for spermatogonia, without attempting to correct for cell killing at this dose.

k This ratio may be taken to indicate the result of extensive differential cell killing, leading to a predominant elimination of cells carrying mutations.

l Pooled data of Russell and Lyon.

Table 2: Values used in calculating expected genetic effects. Linear term α (mutations per locus per R) and quadratic term β (mutations per locus per R^2).

	α term	β term
Maturing oocytes	2.45×10^{-7} ($\pm$ 4.71×10^{-8})	7.79×10^{-10} ($\pm$ 1.13×10^{-10})
Spermatogonia	6.6×10^{-8}	6.7×10^{10}

REFERENCES

[1] Batchelor, A. L., Phillips, R.J.S., and Searle, A.G., Brit J. Radiol. *42*, 448–451 (1969).

[2] BEIR Report, National Academy of Sciences – National Research Council, Washington, D.C. (1972).

[3] Cattanach, B. M. and Moseley, H., Mutation Res. *25*, 63–72 (1974).

[4] Lyon, M.F., Phillips, R.J.S. and Bailey, H.J., Mutation Res. *15*, 185–190 (1972).

[5] Russell, L.B., Mutation Res. *11*, 107–123 (1971).

[6] Russell, W.L., Cold Spring Harbor Symp. Quant. Biol. *16*, 327–336 (1951).

[7] Russell, W.L., Am. Nat. *90*, Suppl. 69–80 (1956).

[8] Russell, W.L., Proc. Natl. Acad. Sci (US) *48*, 1724–1727 (1962).

[9] Russell, W.L., in: Repair from Genetic Radiation Damage (F.H. Sobels ed.) Pergamon Press, Oxford pp. 205–217 (1963).

[10] Russell, W.L., Peaceful Uses of Atomic Energy, 4th 1971 Vol. 13, pp. 487–500 (1972).

[11] Russell, W.L., Russell, L.B., and Kelley, E.M., Science *128*, 1546–1550 (1958).

[12] Searle, A.G., in: Advances in Radiation Biology, Vol. 4 (Lett, J.T., Adler, H. and Zelle, M. eds.) Academic Press, New York pp. 131–207 (1974).

[13] Sobels, F.H., in: Advances Biol. Med. Phys. *12*, 341–352 (1968).

[14] United Nations Scientific Committee on the Effects of Atomic Radiation. Ionizing Radiation: Levels and Effects. Vol. 2 Effects, United Nations, New York (1972).

[15] Wolff, S., in: Annual Review of Genetics, Vol. 1, 221–244 (1967).

CLOSELY LINKED GENES IN THE MAJOR HISTOCOMPATIBILITY COMPLEX (MHC) IN MAN

E. D. ALBERT

Referring to Dr. Legeróva's relevant data on screening for mutations involving the histocompatibility systems in laboratory animals not much is left to add but speculation. In order to provide a basis for speculation I should like to give a brief description of the major histocompatibility complex in man (MHC): The classical histocompatibility antigens (HLA) are cell surface structures defined by serological reactions with alloantisera. Three distinct loci with a series of multiple alleles for each locus have been identified: The first locus (HLA-A, „LA"), the second locus (HLA-B, „FOUR") and the third locus (HLA-C, „AJ") are located on chromosome 6 with a recombination frequency of 0.85 % between HLA-A and HLA-B. HLA-C is located between A and B in close proximity to B.

Considerable crossreactivity has been observed between antigens belonging to the same locus. Absorption-elution experiments have demonstrated that anti-HLA-sera usually contain a number of antibody populations directed against antigenic factors common to several antigens. Absorption and inhibition studies using Fab of such antibody subpopulations have shown that the different crossreacting antibodies combine with different sites of the molecule. The antigenic factors defined by such antibody subpopulations were shown in capping experiments to reside on the same molecule as the respective major HLA antigen. From this information it can be concluded that each HLA antigen possesses a number of antigenic sites of differential immunogenicity. Therefore on the genetic level it must be stressed that within one gene there is information coding for the expression of several different antigenic factors in the same molecule.

The human MHC contains in addition to the above discussed systems of serologically defined (SD) antigens also genes which are responsible for the expression of cell surface structures which elicit a stimulation in mixed leucocyte culture (MLC). The definition of these lymphocyte defined (LD) antigens has been accomplished using cells that could be shown to be homozygous for the MLC allele. One major MLC-locus (HLA-D) is closely linked ($r = 0.98$ %) with the HLA-B locus. Family and population data have provided evidence for the existence of at least one more MLC locus somewhere in the proximity of the HLA-A locus.

Based on the finding of HLA-disease associations is the speculation about HLA-linked disease susceptibility genes which might well be pathologic variants of immune response genes suspected to map in this chromosomal region. More recently linkage has been shown for genes involved in the complement system: The Bf-polymorphism could be located between the HLA-B and HLA-D loci (the Bf-protein acts as the C3-proactivator). The C2 and C4 components are also linked with HLA but their position has not been precisely mapped.

The current concept of the human MHC is schematically summarised as follows:

```
   HLA-A      HLA-E??       HLA-C  HLA-B       Bf       HLA-D
----/---------x-----------/------/-------o--------X---
```

In considering the possibility of monitoring the mutation rate in man using the histocompatibility systems no immediately available and practicable method comes to mind. It is however not impossible that in the future it may become feasable to monitor mutations by an in-vitro-test such as per instance mixed leucocyte culture where minute changes can be detected through the use of surveillance by immuno-competent cells.

SCREENING FOR NEW MUTATIONS AT THE PROTEIN LEVEL. LARGE NUMBER VERSUS SMALL NUMBER OF LOCI TO BE TESTED IN THE INDIVIDUAL: A PROBLEM OF ECONOMY

K. ALTLAND and L. HEREDERO

The principle of a test for mutation rate or change of the latter is to check a certain length of DNA for mutational events. Methods to screen for such events at the level of DNA are not available, and the length of DNA indirectly testable at the protein level is rather small in the individual. Samples of many individuals are therefore needed. The sample size is determined by the number of loci testable in the individual, by the expected mutation rate, and by the required confidence limits of the experimental result.

In recent years many methods have become available to test for mutant individual proteins. The fact, however, that the mutation rate has not been measured using these methods is the consequence of a serious unsolved economic problem: most methods till now are rather unsuitable for screening that is for testing a high number of loci at a low consumption of work and material.

From the paper of Neel and coworkers (1973) it can be calculated that for testing 6.000.000 loci they need 600 person years or 12 minutes* per locus with $^{2}/_{3}$ of this time consumed for collection of samples and $^{1}/_{3}$ for electrophoretic analysis when 20 loci are tested in the individual. Heredero and coworkers (1974) developed an economically optimized electrophoretic screening system for hemoglobins** also suitable for other proteins.

On the basis of economical data obtained with this system for the „best“ 3 loci, e.g. alpha – and beta-chain of hemoglobin and albumin, it should be possible to test the 6.000.000 loci by only 30 person years of work or at a speed of 0.6 minutes per locus, sample collection included. This means $^{1}/_{20}$ of the expense for the 20 protein system of Neel and coworkers.

---

* Calculated on the basis that 1 year = 250 working days of 8 hours = 2,000 hrs.

** The PAA-Gel Screening Electrophoresis System Havana is available from DESAGA, Heidelberg, PO Box 101969

There is no doubt that except for the economical aspect the system of Neel and coworkers has many advantages to that of Heredero et al., the latter being developed for another purpose.
However, the system of Neel et al. appears to remain unrealistic from an economic of view.
Very recently it has been demonstrated by Altland that Vogel's idea to join a screening for fresh mutants in newborns with the already established screening for PKU shows indeed some realistic aspects. Using isoelectric focusing and electrophoresis in PAA-gel individual hemoglobins and albumin could be easily identified in full blood samples dried on filter papers which were sent by mail to a routine PKU laboratory. There is a good chance for testing also other proteins with similar techniques.
It may be concluded that more work on the economical aspect is not only highly needed but also rather promising, and thus will make a monitoring program for mutation rate more easy to perform.

REFERENCES

Heredero, L., Granda, H., Juarez Aguilar, J.A., Altland, K.: Humangenetik 21:167 (1974)

Neel, J.V., Tiffany, T.O., Anderson, N.G. in Hollaender, A. (Ed.): Chemical mutagens. Principles and methods for their detection, Vol. III. Plenum Press. New York – London (1973)

ON THE HETEROZYGOSITY AT THE HL-A GENE LOCI IN CHILDREN AND OLD PEOPLE

K. BENDER

The present study was carried out to contribute to the understanding of the most extensive polymorphism at the HL-A gene loci LA and FOUR (Fig. 1) of the main histocompatibility region (Fig. 2). As to

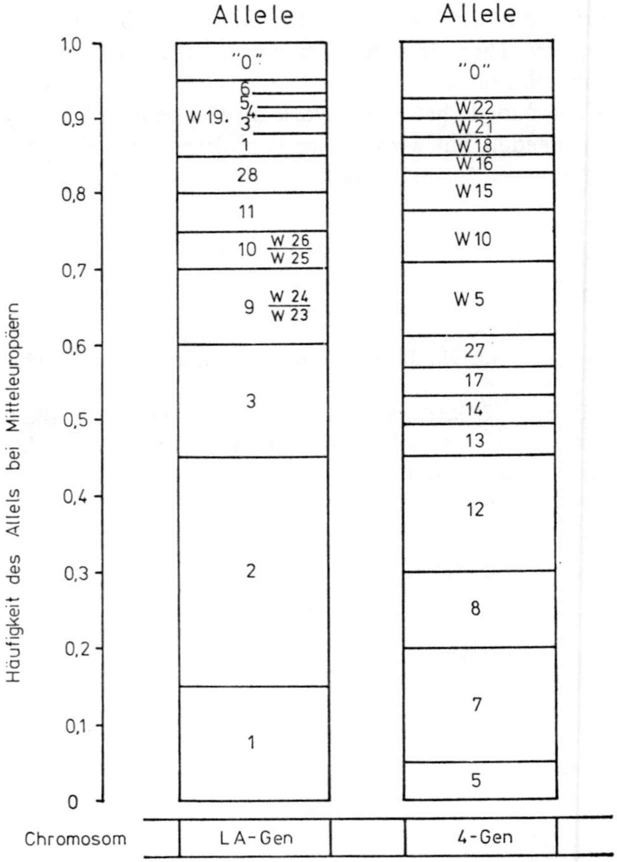

Fig. 1: Formal genetic model of the HL-A system: two closely linked genes, LA and FOUR, both with multiple alleles.

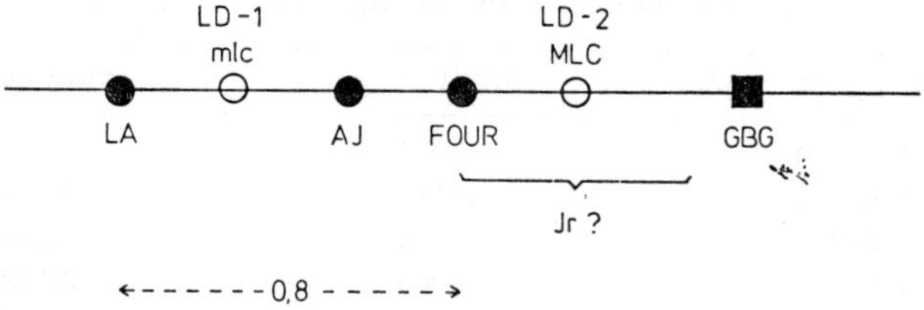

Fig. 2: Representation of the genes of the main human histocompatibility region.

these two genes, three classes of individuals are to be expected, such with 2, 3, and 4 different HL-A antigens. Since HL-A antigens are thought to play an important role in the "self" versus "non self" recognition mechanism, the experiments were based on the following working hypothesis:

1. Heterozygosity at the HL-A loci results in a more "complicated" histocompatibility phenotype than homozygosity, because more different antigenic elements are used to build up the cell surface pattern.
2. Alterations by mutations, oncogenic viruses etc. are monitored more easily by the immune mechanism in "complicated" histocompatibility types than the same alterations in "simple" phenotypes.

According to these assumptions individuals with a high degree of heterozygosity should be equipped with a better surveillance than homozygous persons. Old people who apparently have successfully withstood mutations and neoplastic attacks through all their life should therefore possess a higher degree of heterozygosity than children who have been under this selection pressure for a much shorter period of time.

The data on HL-A allele frequencies as found in 169 children (up to 10 years) and in 182 old people (from 70–93 years) (Table 1), and the frequency distribution of, respectively, 2, 3 and 4 different HL-A antigens (Table 2) revealed, however, no difference between the two population samples. Thus the hypothesis must be rejected.

Table 1: HL-A allele frequencies in 169 children and in 182 people

LA gene	children	old people
HL-A 1	0.1434	0.1518
HL-A 2	0.3119	0.2903
HL-A 3	0.1492	0.1414
HL-A 9	0.1008	0.1096
HL-A10	0.0796	0.1040
HL-A11	0.0586	0.0534
HL-A28	0.0483	0.0339
W19	0.0646	0.0844
X_{LA}	0.0432	0.0308
Four gene		
HL-A 5	0.0485	0.0799
HL-A 7	0.1340	0.1297
HL-A 8	0.1029	0.0644
HL-A12	0.1471	0.1149
HL-A13	0.0414	0.0412
HL-A14	0.0221	0.0329
HL-A17	0.0295	0.0533
HL-A27	0.0591	0.0439
W 5	0.1011	0.1048
W10	0.0891	0.0755
W15	0.0650	0.0671
W16	0.0414	0.0586
W18	0.0532	0.0533
W22	0.0190	0.0302
W21	0.0118	0.0137
X_4	0.0340	0.0357

Table 2: Frequency of occurrence of 2, 3, and 4 different HL-A antigens in 169 children and in 182 old people

Number of different HL-A antigens	Children n	Children %	Old people (70) n	Old people (70) %
4	107	63.3	119	65.4
3	54	32.0	56	30.8
2	8	4.7	7	3.8
	169	100	182	100

$\chi^2 = 0.5 \quad p > 0.90$

During this study a similar work was undertaken by Gerkins et al. (1974). The authors found no homozygous individuals among their healthy old people (all over 75 years of age); they detected, however, a high proportion of homozygous individuals within their samples of young and old cancer patients (Table 3). From these data the authors conclude that HL-A heterozygosity might be a marker of long time survival.

Since the healthy old people in the study of Gerkins et al. (1974) comprised only over 75 years old individuals, we looked at the frequency distribution in our over 75 years old people (Table 3). 120 out of the 182 old individuals belong to this age group. Nevertheless, 4 of them (3,3 %) had only two different HL-A antigens (HL-A2, W15; HL-A1, W5; HL-A2, 12; HL-A9, 7). Thus, the difference between our findings and those of Gerkins et al. (1974) possibly may depend on sampling characteristics. Perhaps the Freiburg populations is more homogeneous than the Los Angeles population.

Table 3: Frequency of occurrence of 2, 3, and 4 different HL-A antigens in the samples of Gerkins et al. (1974) as well as in the > 75 years old Freiburg people

Sample			different HL-A antigens (%)		
		n	4	3	2
Healthy old people (> 75 y)	(Los Angeles)	126	72	28	–
Healthy young (< 36 y)	(Los Angeles)	148	57	36	6
Cancer old people	(Los Angeles)	66	56	4	8
Cancer young	(Los Angeles)	72	64	21	15
Healthy old people (> 75 y)	(Freiburg)	120	66.7	30.0	3.3
Healthy children (< 10 y)	(Freiburg)	169	63.3	32.0	4.7

REFERENCE

Gerkins, V. R., Ting, A., Menck, H. T., Casagrande, J. T., Terasaki, P. I., Pike, M. C., Henderson, B. E.: HL-A heterozygosity as a genetic marker of long time survival. J. Nat. Cancer Inst. 52, 1909–1911 (1974)

EXPERIENCES WITH A MULTIREGIONAL PROSPECTIVE INVESTIGATION ON PREGNANCY COURSE AND CHILD DEVELOPMENT

K. H. DEGENHARDT

The main task of epidemiological studies in the field of congenital defects is the etiological aspect. The detection of true associations between distinct independent and dependent variables concerning single or multiple influencing factors during pregnancy and the outcome of pregnancy resp. the health status of the infant at birth or later on in childhood may allow to state causal relationships. The thalidomide trial in our country threw light on the fact, that our knowledge about harmful environmental events during pregnancy especially with regard to the sensitive period of organogenesis of the fetus seemed to be highly insufficient. Detailed and reliable data about the full load of environmental influencing factors with special attention to the first trimester of pregnancy was urgently needed.

As you know two different approaches are being performed:

retrospective and prospective studies, which may be conducted separately or combined.

A retrospective study starts with the birth of a child with a specified congenital defect. The history of the mother is examined. Events which occured during the critical period of the defective organ may be suspected of being a possible factor in causal relation. The main pitfall of this approach is represented by the possible unreliability of the mother's reply, but we have to keep in mind that the retrospective method already yielded very valuable positive results, i.e. the rubella-embryopathia and the thalidomide embryopathia were detected by this approach.

Prospective investigations exclude any element of bias interest, which predominates in retrospective studies. They start before delivery occurred; usually admission to the study is limited to the first trimester of pregnancy. All data are collected on prepared documentation forms independently from the outcome of pregnancy. This makes the collected data more objective for the recognition of true associations in correlation statistics.

The development of the fetus is the resultant of two main factors:

1. The genetic information contains the programmation of the phenotype of the future child.
2. The environment supplies the nutritients necessary for the growth, cell differentiation and tissue formation in a harmonic equipotential developmental system. Normal development always depends on close interactions between the genome and the normal range of environmental influences. Abnormal development may be evoked by a single gene or a single exogeneous factor; but single events as a cause in the origin of congenital defects seem to be rare in comparison with the large number of birth defects caused by close interrelations between polygenes which constitute a threshold of sensitivity and many different environmental factors.

Concerning the genetic base of congenital defects we also have to consider the strong influence of chromosomal numerical or structural aberrations on developmental processes causing early intrauterine death or characteristic syndromes of structural and functional defects visible at birth or later in childhood.

As it is the aim of the prospective investigation, to deal with the etiology of birth defects, the definition for this determination should be clear. Birth defects are synonym with congenital defects; they consist of abnormalities, both morphological and biochemical, existing before or at birth. They are not necessarily clinically manifest immediately after birth or even during childhood; if detected later in development, they should be attributable to antenatal development uninfluenced by subsequent factors. Congenital malformations signify one subgroup of congenital defects and mean structural defects existing at birth and caused by conditions before birth. The ICD VIII of WHO should be used at least in the 3 digit level as a basis for malformation subcategories; for practical use it has been necessary to modify the ICD list at certain points. Jukka Hakosalo presented valuable recommendations. His nomenclature for subgrouping of congenital defects seems to be quite appropriate for comparison of results in different investigations; he subdivided congenital defects into malformations and functional defects; malformations are subdivided into the generally accepted and the debated malformations. The latter group was considered to comprise those common malformations whose inclusion in the lists presented in the literature is very variable, then affecting the frequency figures significantly, for instance pyloric stenosis, cryptorchism, hydrocele of testis, talipes, dislocation of the hip.

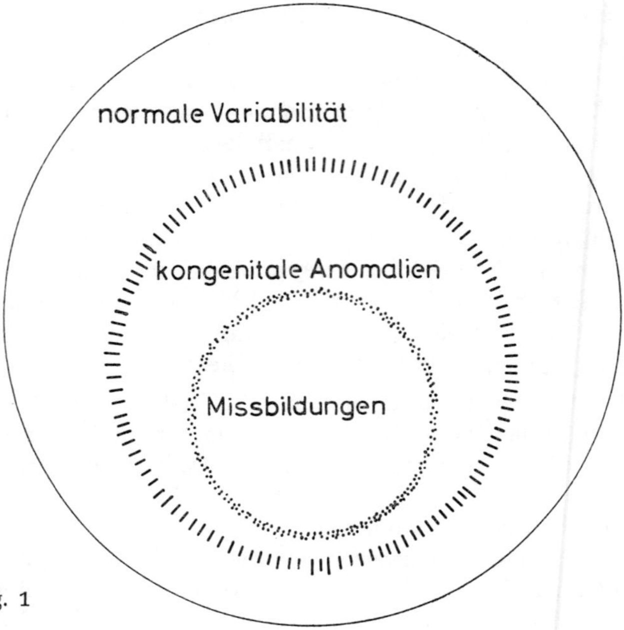

Fig. 1

The aim of the prospective investigation initiated in 1963 by a committee of the German Research Foundation originally was limited to frequencies and etiology of special types of congenital malformations. In the meantime the scope for evaluation has been broadened concerning the outcome of pregnancy and the health status of the newborn and the developing child. A wide spread multiregional collaborative project has been organised together with 18 clinics of obstetrics and gynecology in close cooperation with clinics of pediatrics and special laboratories. The pregnant women, who firstly attended the clinic's precare station because of various reasons, during the first trimester, were asked to join the study. Gynecological reexaminations were performed every 4 weeks. Once in each trimester a blood sample was taken from each woman for examinations on toxoplasmosisantibodies, special virusantibodies (Rubella, Cytomegaly, Mumps) and special serum level distinctions. Special events concerning the health status of the gravida or changes in the private or occupational sphere were recorded in a diary. The collaborating physicians recorded all data in prepared documentation forms; this also concerned the course of

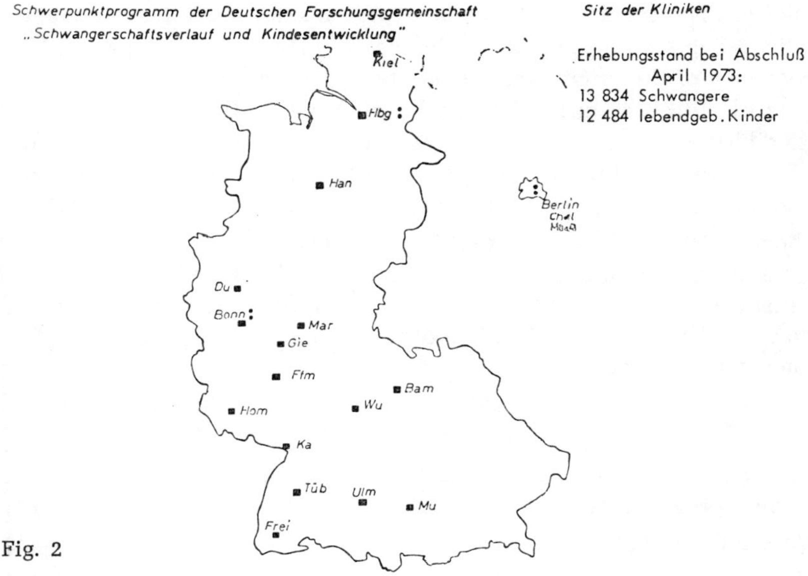

Fig. 2

deliveries and the detailed examinations of the newborn by the obstetrician and by the pediatrician; the children were reexamined four times up to the age of three years. Storing of data and the statistical analysis are being performed by Koller and his colleagues in the department of medical documentation and statistics at Mainz University.

In spring 1973 the clinics of gynecology and obstetrics finished their collaboration; the clinics of pediatrics continue reexaminations of the children until spring 1976.

Up to now 13.834 pregnancies were registered. 12.210 pregnancies resulted in single livebirth (88.3 %), 116 pregnancies had single stillbirths (0.8 %). Multiple births were seen in the outcome of 140 pregnancies (137 pairs of twins and 3 triplets with 274 livebirths and 10 stillbirths). Spontaneous abortions were registered in the outcome of 1344 pregnancies (9.7 %). 7 twin abortions were seen.

In collecting data on pregnancy special attention was focussed on the living conditions and habits of the women and socioeconomic factors concerning the husband.

The population studied may be selected. For instance there is a higher frequency of gravidas with planned children than in the general population. The age distribution was appr. the same as in the general statistics of the whole population in the German Federal Republic. The frequency of the primiparae seemed to be higher. Appr. equal were the rates of stillbirths and infants, who died within the first seven days after birth (PU 2.9 %). The motivation of the first attendance of the gravidas in the clinic was in at least 75 % the diagnosis of pregnancy; in about 2.3 % the women were in observation because of sterility.

About 4.500 variables were registered for each pregnancy and the outcome including child's development up to three years of age. For statistical evaluations 450 variables were chosen. The frequencies of the variables were described in a cohort of about 6.100 pregnancies. Some examples may be presented here:

	%	h
Wanted pregnancies	67.1	4105
Women beyond 35 years of age	7.2	440
History of the family with diabetes	7.1	434
History with disease of CNS	2.1	131
History with congenital malformations	1.6	99
Preceeding pregnancies with abortions and stillbirth	16.0	1008
Pregnancies with known conception by basal temperature	6.3	388
Outcome with major congenital malformations	1.7	101
Outcome with minor congenital malformations	15.5	947

Some preliminary evaluations may be discussed concerning

- The effects of diabetes in pregnancy
- The effects of bleeding early in pregnancy
- The possible effects of some socio-economic factors
- The effects of paternal smoking habits
- The effects of anticonvulsants and of sex hormones.

There are some preliminary prospectively collected data concerning diabetes and the outcome of pregnancy. In a collective of 8.015 pregnancies the incidence of diabetes was appr. 1 %. The outcome of pregnancies in diabetic women was as follows:

		Controls
live born healthy children	69.2 %	79.0 %
perinatal mortality rate	11.1 %	2.7 %
spontaneous abortions	16.1 %	12.2 %
major congen. malformation	5.0 %	1.8 %

The differences in comparison with the control group are quite obvious. In the group of diabetic women 4 infants with major congen. malformations were seen: in one case a leftsided threefold lung lobation, in two cases congenital heart defects, in one case multiple congen. malformations. The latter case may be of special interest. The mother was 29 of age and a 3rd para. Diabetes has been detected during the 8th week of pregnancy. At once dietary restrictions were ordered and insulin was applied 15–20 IU daily. Delivery had been induced 4 weeks before term. The liveborn child was asphyctic and died at the age of 8 weeks. The following malformations were registered: A large omphalocele with ileum eventration, coecum and colon were rudimentary, the bladder was exstrophic, analatresia, rudimentary external male genitalia, a broad median cleft of the anterior pelvic girdle, axial defects, a syndactyly between the toes III and IV on the left. There seems to be no question, that the heavy imbalance in glucose metabolism may have damaged the embryo in a quite early sensitive period of organogenesis.

Outcome of pregnancy and severe malformations in 8015 diabetic and non-diabetic women

outcome	diabetic	non-diabetic
normal	69,2 %	79,0 %
unknown	2,5 %	4,3 %
abortion	16,1 %	12,2 %
perinatal mortality	11,1 %	2,7 %
severe malformations	5,0 %	1,8 %

(* 3,9 % with severe malformations added)

trimenon 1st	2nd	3rd	%
—	—	—	87,9
+	+	+	2,1
—	+	+	4,9
—	—	+	4,1
+/—	+/—	+/—	1,0

Glucosuria in pregnancy (+) of 5239 women

The incidence of glucosuria could be defined in a collective of 5.239 pregnant women, using a papertest from Boehringer. It amounted to 12.1 %, but only 2.1 % of the pregnant women showed glucosuria in all three trimesters of pregnancy. The incidence increased with the ongoing pregnancy, but also with the age of the women. These observations confirm data, which have been reported from different research groups in various countries.

The significance of glucosuria in relation to the health status of the mother and to the outcome of pregnancy is not yet clear. The glucose

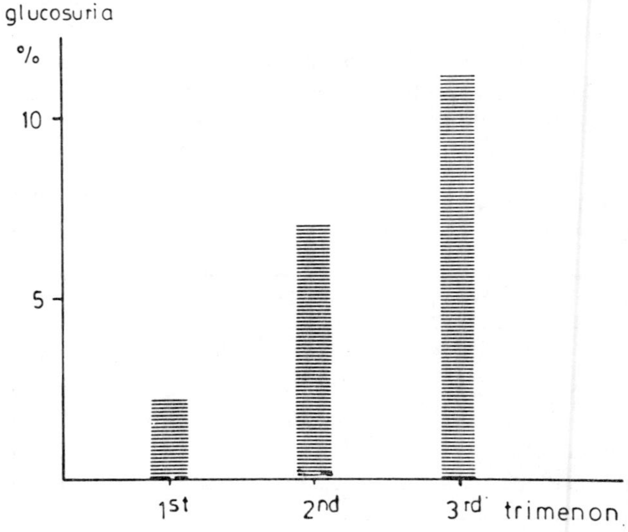

Fig. 3: Frequency of glucosuria in the course of 5239 pregnancies

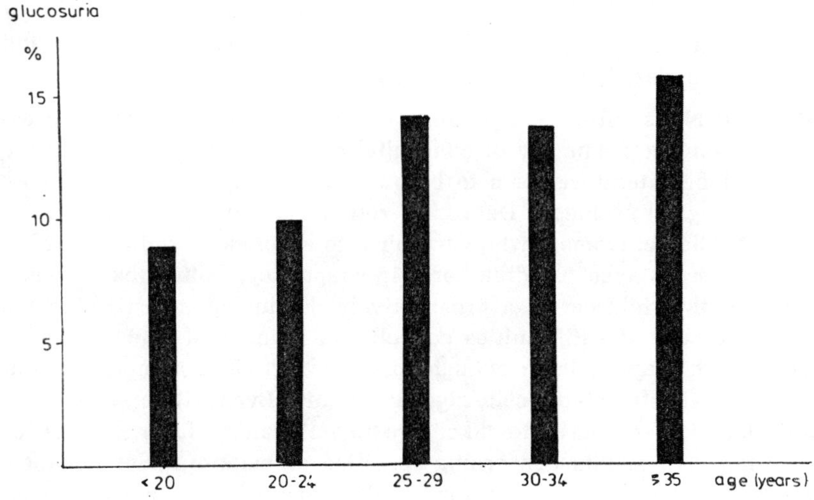

Fig. 4: Frequency of glucosuria corresponding to age in 4422 women

tolerance test and the insulin blood serum level would be conveniant methods to detect causal relationships. But these testsystems have not been used in all participating clinics regularly.

A special investigation is being performed by Staffeldt at Berlin Free University, clinic of gynecology and obstetrics.

Staffeldt performed the glucose tolerance test intravenously and defined the insulin bloodserum level in 317 prospectively registered pregnant women during the 3rd trimester. He stated:

Glucose assimilation was diminished significantly in pregnant women of normal weight but with diabetic relatives of the 1st degree, in pregnant women who gave birth to a child with overweight (4000 g), or to a dead infant and in pregnant women with overweight.

Insulin serum level was dimished in pregnant women with infants, who had overweight; in addition they had a significantly increased preprandial glucose level. There seems to be a true correlation between overweight of the newborn and a decreased function of alpha and beta cells in the Langerhan's islets of the pancreas. The increased preprandial blood glucose serum level causes a higher supply of glucose for the fetus; this may disturb developmental processes and may lead to disrailments in certain sensitive organanlagen.

Mau and Netter discussed possible effects of bleeding early in pregnancy upon the frequency of congenital malformations. Reports in the international literature seem to be quite controverse. There are many methodological problems. Data from retrospectively performed studies are not reliable; women, who gave birth to a defective child remember events, for instance bleeding early in pregnancy, better than women with healthy children. In a prospectively conducted investigation we are faced with the difficulties collecting a number of pregnancies at term which may be large enough to get a sufficient number of congenital defects for statistically significant data. Even with prospectively collected data we have to take care in not getting false positive or false negative results concerning specified associations. For instance, if we correlate the variables for bleeding in pregnancy and perinatal mortality we may have a significant but false positive association because of the fact that both variables are significantly related to prematurity resp. duration of pregnancy. If we correlate bleeding with perinatal mortality in cases of women with infants of the same duration of pregnancy no association may be stated anymore.

Age in years	Perin. + in %	Preterm ($\leqq$ 260 d) in %	of n	% Age Distrib.
< 20	1,6 (0,4)	9,3	256	4,9
20–25	2,3 (0,6)	8,1	1 369	26,3
25–30	3,1 (0,8)	9,3	2 168	41,6
30–35	5,0 (0,9)	10,7	1 085	20,8
> 35	4,5 (1,0)	13,9	332	6,4
Summary	3,3 (0,8)	9,6	5 210	100,0
X^2	$p < 1$ %	$p < 5$ %	–	–

The same is true concerning the age of the women. Though bleeding and congenital malformations in infants of elder women seemed to be more frequent, the true association could be due to the age af the women. Therefore women of the same age may not show any relation between bleeding and congenital malformations.

A quite convenient method in the analysis of true correlations is the technique of matched pairs resp. triples; i.e. for each case of pregnancy resulting in a child with a congenital malformation one or two cases out of the total collective may be chosen being identical in defined control variables with the cases whose pregnancies resulted in congenital malformations.

The hypothesis should be tested whether the two collectives show differences in relation to frequency and time of occurence of bleeding. Analysis has been performed in a collective of 5.000 pregnancies. Incidence of bleeding during the pregnancies up to month 4 was 21 %. 80 pregnancies which resulted in infants with relatively severe congenital malformations were chosen out of the total collective; for each case two control cases were matched concerning the age of the woman, duration of pregnancy, parity and number of previous abortions. The definition of major congenital malformation seems to be quite clear, because we deal with heavy structural and functional congenital defects, but in reality the limitation to minor congenital structural defects may be quite arbitrary and subjective. But this does not much influence the relevant analysis, because the control cases were indeed pregnancies with quite healthy children. The comparison of the two collectives did not show differences in the frequency of bleedings in the early pregnancies. Even in the case of comparison concerning the bleeding time in pregnancy the distribution of bleedings up to 4 months of pregnancy was equal in both collectives.

These statements are valid only with reservations because of the possibility that other not yet detected influencing factors may be responsible.

Recently Mau and Netter, a pediatrician and a statistician of our group analysed the possible effects of some socio-economic factors during pregnancy upon the perinatal death rate, the rate of prematurity and some other perinatal variables.

It is well known that the perinatal death rate depends also on the social status of the parents, i. e. it increases with a lower social status. Up to now we don't know much about single factors of the socio-economic environment which influence the perinatal period. In this special evaluation preliminary results are based on approx. 5.500 pregnancies. Three different kinds of variables were chosen:

1. *Potential influencing factors*
   This includes the occupational sphere (kind and duration of employment, daily duty hours, piece work, assembly line work, carrying heavy loads, ionizing rays or smoke molestation) and it includes the private sphere (daily working time within the home and in the garden, carrying heavy loads, sports, sleeping depth and sleeping time).

The second kind of variables concern dependent factors,
i.e. perinatal death, duration of pregnancy, birth weight and placental weight and the APGAR score.

The third kind of variables are control factors,
i.e. age of the parents, parity, occupation of the husband, family status.

Parity	Perin. + in %	Preterm in %	of n	% Distrib.
No child	3,0	8,7	2488	47,3
1 child	2,7	8,9	1859	35,4
Several child.	5,0	13,7	911	17,3
Summary	3,3	9,6	5258	100,0
X^2	$p < 1\,\%$	$p < 1\,\%$	–	–

Fam. Status	Perin. + in %	Preterm in %	of n	% Distrib.
Unmarried	4,4	14,7	68	1,3
Married bec. of Pregnancy	2,5	7,0	359	7,0
Married	3,3	9,6	4696	91,4
Widow/Divorced	(13)	(27)	15	0,3
Summary	3,3	9.6	5138	100,0
X^2	$p > 5\,\%$	$p < 5\,\%$	–	–

Patern. Occupat.	Perin. + in %	Preterm in %	of n	% Distrib.
Independent	4,1	10,8	530	10,3
Civil Serv.	2,9	7,6	746	14,5
Employee	2,8	9,3	1904	37,1
Worker	3,8	10,9	1662	32,3
Student	3,0	7,1	296	5,8
Summary	3,3	9,6	5138	100,0
X^2	$p > 5\%$	$p < 10\%$	–	–

First of all the potential influencing factors were checked against different groups of age and parity of the mother and against different groups of paternal occupation. Furtheron the dependance upon the family status has been tested. In this descriptive part of evaluation, checking the control variables against the dependent traits, the following observations were made:

1. With increasing maternal age the rate of premature newborn goes up and causes a higher rate of perinatal deaths.
2. The same is true concerning higher parity, which is closely related to higher age.
3. With regard to paternal occupation, prematurity and perinatal death rate were highest in the group of the independents and the workers.
4. The influence of the family status seems to be most unfavourable in the group of the unmarried and the widows resp. divorced. Remarkably low is the rate of premature birth and stillbirth in the group of women, who conceived unmarried but got married because of pregnancy.

The examination of correlation between maternal occupational influencing factors and mentioned dependent variables resulted in two interesting relations, significant only on the 5 % level.

Pregnant women with already one child not involved in occupation had a lower rate of premature and dead newborn than those women who were employed. The opposite was true in women who had their first pregnancy, i.e. the lower rate of prematurity and death was in the group of women with employment; but here the higher rate of risk pregnancies was in the group of women, who stayed at home and did not work outside because of the risk. Comparison of the two groups

with and without employment during pregnancy without a prior child seemed to be quite limited because of the unequal distribution of risk pregnancies.
Similar difficulties concerning comparison were seen in testing the other occupational variables, i.e. early duty hours and duration of them, piece work and assembly line work. It was obvious that women with risk pregnancies for instance usually work less hours daily and give up their employent much earlier.

Employment	Perin. + in %	Preterm in %	of n
No	2,1	8,0	1051
Yes	3,6	9,8	798
Summary	2,8	8,8	1849
X^2	p 5 %	5 %	–

Working Position	Perin. + in %	Preterm $\leq$ 260 d. in %	Birthweight $\leq$ 2500 g in %	of n
Sitting	2,6	8,5	5,2	879
Standing	5,5	11,4	9,9	473
Changing	4,3	8,5	8,0	626
Summary	38	92	72	1978
X^2	$p < 5$ %	> 5 %	< 5 %	–

The quality of the working place with regard to sitting, running, standing or changing position showed a more reliable result in comparison with the different groups of pregnant women.
It could be seen that pregnant women with a sitting position in their employment are favoured because of the lower rate of premature and dead newborn. In the group of pregnant women with standing working condition the incidences of premature and dead newborn were highest.
This relation could not be stated in the group of official dependents or in the age group of the 25–30, which contains a quite increased number of women of official dependents. Under this aspect we should

be very reserved to call the relation between a special working condition and perinatal variables true ones because other factors not yet detected could be involved.
Concerning the private sphere no relations could be found to the above mentioned dependent variables.
Performing a comprehensive analysis about the influence of food and luxury consumption during pregnancy, Mau and Netter stated a quite remarkable correlation between paternal smoking habits and an increased perinatal death rate.
The interims report is based on appr. 5.200 pregnancies at term with a perinatal death rate of 3.3 % as a consequence of a slightly increased number of risk pregnancies in the study group. This selection is not of importance because comparisons are made within the prospectively collected data.
Smoking habits of the husbands were as follows:

49.7 % did not smoke
20.9 % smoked 1–10 cigarettes daily
29.4 % smoked more than 10 cigarettes daily.

For the analysis of incidences X^2 test has been used. To exlude paternal age influence, the expected values have been standardised with concern to age distribution.
Perinatal death rate was significantly increased in the group of husbands smoking more than 10 cigarettes daily. This is also true with regard to pregnant women who did not smoke.
The possible influence of 11 other variables could be ruled out; i.e. single clinic effect, age of mother, number of preceding pregnancies, abortions and stillbirth, occupation of father, study and treatment because of sterility.

The detailed analysis of possible causes and conditions of perinatal mortality gave the following results:

1. The frequency of stillbirth increases with heavier paternal smoking habits (significance below 1 %).
2. The frequency of major congenital malformations is increased in infants of husbands with heavier smoking habits. Maternal smoking habits did not influence this correlation. The increase of perinatal mortality was independent from the incidence of major congenital malformation at birth. With other words the increase of incidence of major congenital malformations was clearly seen in infants who survived.

The correlation between paternal smoking habits and the increased incidence of congenital malformations was independent from the parent's age, social status and individual clinic. Association between daily paternal smoking habits and specified types of malformations were not sure, but facial clefts and multiple malformations are obviously frequent.

The rate of spontaneous abortions was not significantly increased in dependence upon paternal smoking habits.

The causes of the above mentioned associations concerning perinatal mortality and major congenital malformations are not yet clear. We may think of mutagenic effects of substances within the cigarette smoke, i.e. Benzpyren. The effects may be different on paternal and maternal germs because of the very different reproductive capacities.

Paternal Cigarettes Consumption and Major Congen. Malformations

Cigarettes daily	Major congen. malformations in %	of n
No cigarettes	0,8	2563
1–10	1,4	1089
> 10	2,1	1509
Summary	1,3	5161

$X^2 = 12{,}4$, $P < 1\,\%$

Paternal Cigarettes Consumption and Perinatal Mortality

Cigarettes daily	Perin. mortality in %	of n
No cigarettes	3,0 (1,3)	2575
1–10	2,5 (0,8)	1085
> 10	4,5 (1,6)	1523
Summary	3,3 (1,3)	5183

$X^2 = 10{,}4$, $P < 1\,\%$

Several investigators reported on a positive correlation between paternal smoking habits and incidence of abnormal spermatozoa.
We should not yet claim the correlations true ones until other investigators could confirm this in epidemiological or experimental studies.
In May 1973 Jean Fredrik, research epidemiologist at the University of Oxford, reported on a retrospectively performed investigation concerning epilepsy and pregnancy. The files of the Oxford Record Linkage Study were used to identify 223 infants delivered to 168 epileptic women as the result of 218 pregnancies. There were 6 stillbirth, two of which were grossly malformed, i.e. 2.69 % in comparison with 1.06 % among the 71.000 total deliveries to women resident in the area over a five year period. There were highly significant excesses of congenital defects among the infants born to epileptic mothers, i.e. 13.8 % of livebirths had some degree of a congenital defect compared with 5.6 % of controls. The mothers ascertained as epileptic in the Oxford area differed in their age and social class distribution from the total maternity population. Both factors have some influence on the incidence of congenital defects. Therefore it is imperative for comparison that the controls have the same distribution. Even when the controls were matched for social class, maternal age and parity, there were more than twice as many congenital defects among the livebirths delivered to epileptic mothers – both considering those identified at birth and those recognized later in childhood up to the age of five years.
It was shown that neither the frequency with which the mother had fits nor the length of time she had had the epilepsy seemed to bear any relation to the frequency of congenital defects in the offspring. There appeared to be a dosage effect with phenobarbitone but not with phenytoin. The observed spectrum of congenital defects did not show any preference of a special type.
Some preliminary data are available in our prospective study concerning epilepsy, use of anticonvulsants and outcome of pregnancy. In a collective of 10.360 pregnancies 23 epileptic woman with 27 pregnancies were registered. It would have been ideal to compare a group of epileptic women with and without intake of an anticonvulsant to separate the influences of the disease and the drug. But this could not be done; one epileptic woman only did not use anticonvulsants during pregnancy; she gave birth to a healthy child. This evaluation

Anticonvulsants in Pregnant Epileptic Women

Group of Pregnancies	Outcome of Pregnancies* Abortion	Stillbirth	Livebirth < 260 d	Livebirth > 260 d	Summary
Epileptic Women	4 (15,4 %)	–	1 (3,8 %)	21 (80,8 %)	26 (100,0 %)
Matched Controls	5 (9,6 %)	–	2 (3,9 %)	45 (86,5 %)	52 (100,0 %)
					–
					78

* out of 10,360 prospect. reg. pregnancies

is based on the outcome of 26 pregnancies of 22 epileptic women. To each of these pregnancies two control cases were matched for maternal age, outcome of preceding pregnancies, week of pregnancy for admission to the study and the individual clinic. Ten different anticonvulsant drugs were used, predominantly diphenylhydantoin (19 x), 8 women ingested one special drug, 14 women used 2 or 3 different anticonvulsants at the same time.

Eleven epileptic women ingested additional drugs, i.e. Valium, sex hormones. In spite of the anticonvulsant therapy 12 women had convulsions during pregnancy, in one case petit mal fits.

The only differences to the matched control cases could be seen in the abortion and malformation rates, but the numbers are too small to assure this. Congenital malformations were seen in 3 infants in each of the two groups. In the group of epileptic mothers 22 livebirths were registered; the congenital defects could be defined as follows:

one infant with a mild microcephaly and some physical peculiarities (left lid aperture and left ear smaller, brachycephaly, naevi flammei), a second infant with atrioventricular defects of the heart, a third infant with a slight hypospady.

In the control group of 47 infants the following congenital defects were seen: One infant with the so called Rubinstein syndrom (broad thumbs and big toes, a characteristic dysplastic face and mental retardation), the second infant had a congenital dislocation of the hip, the third infant showed a turricephaly and additional physical dysplastic signs.

No differences could be found concerning the duration of pregnancy, the birth weight of the infants, the Apgar score after 5 minutes. There may be an increase of neurological signs during the period of the newborns in the group of infants of epileptic mothers, i.e. trembling, tremor, excitements; but these signs are transitional. Examinations in development of early childhood up to the age of three years presented normal function of the CNS, except in the child with microcephaly.

We should be very reserved to draw conclusions from these observations. The increase of abortions and congenital defects in the group of epileptic mothers has to be confirmed with larger numbers of prospectively registered epileptic pregnant women.

PREGNANCIES AT TERM: 8,874

INFANTS with

ascertained HEART DEFECTS: 33 = 0.37 %

inclusive transposition of great vessels 4 = 0.0045 %

In 1973 Levy, Nora and Oakley independently reported on possible relations between application of oestrogens and gestagens early in pregnancy and the incidence of congenital heart defects specified as transpositions of the great vessels. Koller and Michaelis stated 33 infants with ascertained congenital heart defects in a collective of 8874 prospectively registered pregnancies at term. 4 cases of transposition of great vessels could be verified. Only 13 out of the 33 women, whose pregnancy resulted in a child with congenital heart defect had intake of sex hormones (= 39 %), i.e. 5 women performed a pregnancy test with duogynon and 8 women ingested other sex hormones. The analysis using the matched pair technique with 66 control cases without congenital malformations resulted in the following observations: 16 of 66 women ingested sex hormones, i.e. 6 woman had a pregnancy test with duogynon, 9 women had intake of other sex hormones. 50 pregnant women did not use any hormone. Only in one of 4 cases of transposition of great vessels, the pregnant mother had intake of gestanon during the 7. – 8. week. This means, we cannot confirm an association between sex hormones and transposition of great vessels. There seems to be an increase of sex hormone intake in the group of women with infants who presented congenital heart defects in comparison with control cases; but the difference is not significant.

Drug	Heart Defects: Total	Heart Defects: Transposition of great Vessels	Matched Controls without congen. malform.
Duogynon^R	5 (15.2 %)	0	6 (9.1 %)
Contraceptiva	0 (0 %)	0	1 (1.5 %)
Other Sex Hormones	8 (24.2 %)	1 (Gestanon^R) 7/8 wks preg.	9 (13.6 %)
No Sex Hormones	20 (60.6 %)	3 (1*)	50 (75.8 %)
Infants	33 (100.0 %)	4 (5*)	66 (100.0 %)

* One case not ascertained by autopsy

May I summarize my impressions also in the light of many critical discussions we had at the 3rd meeting of the European Teratology Society in Helsinki with our colleagues:

We should use the many various methodological approaches to enlighten and unravel the serious problems with concern to the etiology of congenital defects, i.e. we should intensify our efforts with regard to retrospective and prospective epidemiological studies. The disadvantages of prospectively performed investigations are quite obvious:

High financial budgets were needed and the long term studies are a real psychological problem. The advantages of this kind of study are: More reliable data about environmental influences especially during the early period of pregnancy and the fact that the controls are much easier at hand. This may help to understand the importance of the influences of various drugs as well as the occupational and the private spheres in their full load of harm to the ongoing pregnancy. We have to take into account the fact that most of congenital defects are due to a close interrelationship between the genome and a distinct environmental situation. The first step of disrailment in any case is a subcellular biochemical dysfunction followed by irreversible morphological changes; this may be on the basis of a lowered threshold in certain organanlagen caused by several genes.

REFERENCES

Hakosalo, J.K.: Cumulative detection rates of congenital malformation in a ten-year follow-up study Acta Pathol.Microbiol.Scand. Sec. A (1973) Suppl. No. 242

Staffeldt, K.: Glukosetoleranz und Insulinsekretion in der Schwangerschaft bei potentiellem Diabetes mellitus. Habilitationsschrift, Freie Universität Berlin (1971)

Mau, G., Netter, P.: Blutungen in der Frühschwangerschaft – ein Hinweis auf kindliche Mißbildungen? Z.Kinderheilk. 117, 79–88 (1974)

Mau, G., Netter, P., Knörr, K.: Socio-ökonomische Faktoren in der Schwangerschaft und ihre Auswirkungen auf perinatale Sterblichkeit, Frühgeburtlichkeit und andere perinatale Größen. In: Perinatale Medizin V, 16–17 (J.W. Dudenhausen u. E. Saling Hrsg.) Thieme Stuttgart (1974)

Mau, G., Netter, P.: Auswirkungen des väterlichen Zigarettenkonsums auf die perinatale Sterblichkeit und Mißbildungshäufigkeit. Dtsch.Med.Wschr. 99, 1113–1118 (1974)

Fedrick, J.: Epilepsy and Pregnancy: A Report from the Oxford Record Linkage Study. Br.Med.J. 2, 442–448 (1973)

Levy, E.P., Cohen, A., Fraser, F.C.: Hormone treatment during pregnancy and congenital heart defects. Lancet I, 611 (1973)

Nora, J.J., Nora, A.H.: Birth Defects and Oral Contraceptives. Lancet I, 941–942 (1973)

Oakley, G.P. and Flynt, J.W.: Hormonal pregnancy tests and congenital malformations. Lancet II, 256 (1973)

Koller, S., Michaelis, H.: personal communication

A NEW TYPE OF GENETICALLY DETERMINED DISEASES: HORMONE RECEPTOR DEFECTS*

WOLFGANG ENGEL and JOACHIM FROWEIN

The garden-dwarf and the African pygmies

The garden dwarf was thought to be a typical german invention. According to Quiring (1948) and Goebert (1974) the garden-dwarf seems to have a mythological or even historical basis, namely the so called "dactyls" or "fingermen", an indogermanic tribe which inhabited Crete 2000 years ago. The dactyls were of extremely short stature and they were engaged in the prospecting for ore and the production of various metals, especially gold and silver. According to the above mentioned authors the dactyls might have performed extensive expeditions covering most parts of Europe, including Germany.

A recent example of a human population which is characterized by an extreme, but proportionate shortness of stature are the African pygmies. Because of their resemblance to persons with isolated growth hormone deficiency, it has been suggested that African pygmies' short stature is due to a genetic defect resulting in growth hormone deficiency (Kupperman, 1963). However, normal plasma concentrations of unaltered human growth hormone (HGH) have been demonstrated (Rimoin et al., 1967). It may therefore be assumed that the pygmies exhibit a peripheral subresponsiveness to the hormonal action of HGH, possibly caused by a hormone receptor defect (Rimoin et al., 1969). Shortness of stature in the pygmies might be due to a single gene mutation which is present in all individuals of the population.

Hormones and some characteristics of their receptors

Hormones can be classified into two groups, namely the steroid hormones like testosterone, estrogen and cortisol on the one side and the polypeptide hormones like growth hormone, follicle stimulating hormone and luteinizing hormone on the other side. Hormones are

* This work was supported by the Deutsche Forschungsgemeinschaft (Sonderforschungsbereich 46)

produced by the endocrine organs and transported by the blood and the lymphstream to all cells of the organism.

However, the biological activity of any hormone is restricted to specific cells and organs, so-called target cells or target organs. The absolute prerequisite for a cell to function as a target cell for a definite hormone is the presence of the specific receptor. Receptors are characterized by high specifity and high affinity to their respective hormone. Nonresponsiveness or subresponsiveness of a target organ to its hormone point to a hormone receptor defect.

Steroid hormones and their interaction with target cells

Steroid hormones enter the cell by diffusion and are bound to cytoplasmic receptors. Steroid hormone receptors are allosteric proteins. According to their sedimentation behaviour in sucrose gradients defined by ionic strength, mainly three different receptor molecules can be found in the cell: 3–4 S, 5–6 S and 8–10 S. The steroid hormone associates with a 8 S receptor, which is a tetrameric molecule. This 8 S hormone receptor complex (HRC) dissociates into a 4 S HRC, which seems to be a dimeric molecule, and into various other nonhormone-binding subunits. In a temperature dependent step the 4 S HRC is transformed into a 5 S HRC („transformation"), which is then translocated into the nucleus („translocation") and there bound to specific acceptor sites in the chromatin or possibly to DNA. Only the 5 S-HRC is biologically active, specifically influencing the activity of the genome. The steroid hormone-target cell interaction is schematically demonstrated in Figure 1.

Steroid hormone receptor defects:
Testicular feminization and some further candidates

In accordance with Figure 1, steroid hormone receptor defects should be caused by disturbances on different levels of the hormone receptor interaction. This assumption is supported by the results of investigations on the glucocorticoid sensitivity of mouse lymphoma cells in culture. Normally, these cells express a glucocorticoid receptor and, in consequence, are lysed in the presence of the hormone. Using selective media with 10^{-7} M dexamethasone, glucocorticoid resistant lymphoma cells have been found, in which the insensitivity to the hormone is due to different receptor defects. In 80 % of the cells the cytoplasmic

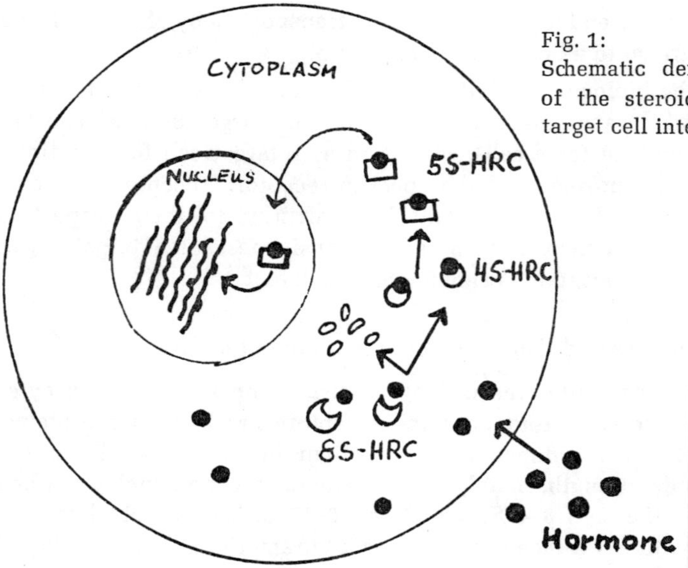

Fig. 1:
Schematic demonstration of the steroid hormone-target cell interaction

receptor was lacking, in 10 % the cells were deficient in the transfer of the hormone-receptor complex to nuclei, while in the remaining 10 % of the resistant cells the 5 S HRC could not be bound to the chromatin (Sibley and Tomkins, 1974; Gehring and Tomkins, 1974). From these results it can be inferred that a considerable genetic heterogeneity may underlie to "steroid hormone receptor defects".

Till now only one genetic defect has clearly been shown to be caused by a steroid hormone receptor defect. This is testicular feminization (Tfm) in man (Keenan et al., 1974), mouse (Attardi and Ohno, 1974; Gehring and Tomkins, 1974) and rat (Bullock and Bardin, 1972; Milin and Roy, 1973). A mutation leading to a very similar phenotype has also been observed in cattle (Short, 1967). The affected individuals exhibit a female phenotype while their sex chromosome constitution is XY. Uterus, oviducts and ovaries are lacking while there are small abdominal testes. In the Tfm-mouse all target cells of androgens are totally unresponsive to testosterone and 5α-dihydrotestosterone. Affected target organs include: embryonic Wolffian ducts and urogenital sinus, hypothalamus-pituitary axis, kidney proximal tubules, submaxillary glands and mammary glands (see reviews by Ohno, 1971; 1974). Androgen insensitivity during embryonal development in XY-fetus leads to the regression of the Wolffian ducts, which are the anlage of the secondary male sex organs. In consequence, the XY-fetus develops a female phenotype.

Androgen insensitivity in man, mouse and rat is exclusively caused by the lack of cytoplasmic androgen receptors. However, in man a significant amount of clinical heterogeneity among unrelated individuals with testicular feminization has been described (Wilkins, 1965; Boczkowski, 1971). This might be due to different mutations at the Tfm-gene locus or even at different gene loci resulting in a similar situation as described for the glucocorticoid resistant mouse lymphoma cells (Sibley and Tomkins, 1974; Gehring and Tomkins, 1974).

In man and mouse the Tfm-gene locus is proven to be X-linked (Lyon and Hawkes, 1970; Meyer et al., 1975). Present knowledge of gene mapping in mammals suggests that all mammalian X-chromosomes carry the same genes (Ohno, 1973). It may therefore be assumed that also in rat, cattle and any other mammal testicular feminization is due to an X-linked hormone receptor defect.

Other defects which might be caused by steroid hormone receptor defects are: Del Pozos type of pseudohypogonadism for testosterone (Del Pozo, 1972), and cases of idiopathic respiratory distress syndrome in newborns for glucocorticoids (Ballard and Ballard, 1972).

Polypeptide hormones and their interactions with target cells

In contrast to steroid hormones the biological activity of polypeptide hormones is transmitted into the target cells by a specific receptor present *in* the cell membrane. As an example, in the male luteinizing hormone (LH) can only affect the Leydig cells of the testis because these cells are the only ones exhibiting an LH hormone receptor. Binding of the hormone to the receptor results in a stimulation of a receptor associated enzyme, adenyl cyclase. In consequence of this, the production of cyclic adenosine 3', 5'-monophosphate (cAMP) is increased. cAMP acts at different intracellular levels, obviously also by inducing genetic activity.

Defects possibly due to polypeptide hormone receptor defects

Polypeptide hormone receptor defects are discussed to be responsible for the following defects, which have partially been observed to be familiarly transmitted.

- Pseudohypoparathyroidism (for references see below),
- Nephrogenic diabetes insipidus (Fichman and Brooker, 1972; Schultz and Lines, 1975),
- Insensitivity to human growth hormone (Rimoin et al., 1969), thyreotrophin (Stanbury et al., 1968),
  and adrenocorticotrophic hormone (Kelch et al., 1972),
- Kallmann syndrome (Bardin et al., 1969),
- Gonadotrophin resistant ovary syndrome (Kim, 1974),
- Fertile eunuch syndrome (Bonati et al., 1974),
- Diabetes in older age.

Of these, pseudohypoparathyroidism is the most extensively investigated defect. Affected individuals have abnormally high blood concentrations of parathyroid hormone, and the secretion of the hormone responds normally to the physiological control by calcium. However, the target organs including bones and kidney are unresponsive to the hormone (Chase et al., 1969). The patients exhibit hypocalcemia, short stature and various malformations of the bones. Injections of parathyroid hormone is ineffective (Chase et al., 1969), while after treatment with cAMP, calcium mobilization in the bones as well as urinary phosphate clearance, markedly increased, 30 to 50 fold (Bell et al., 1972). According to these results pseudohypoparathyroidism is very likely caused by a parathyroid hormone receptor defect.

Other receptor defects and concluding remarks

Myasthenia gravis is a neuromuscular disorder, characterized by muscular weakness and fatigability, especially for the muscles of the eyes and the face. Although the abnormality is known to involve the neuromuscular junction, the precise nature of the defect is still uncertain. However, Fambrough et al., (1973) have shown recently that in neuromuscular junctions of myasthenic muscles the number of acetylcholine receptors was 80–90 % lower as compared to controls. This reduction in receptor concentration may account for the defect in the neuromuscular transmission in myasthenia gravis.

Receptor defects are also under discussion in the familiarly transmitted refractoriness to thyroid hormone (Refetoff et al., 1967) and in juvenile diabetes for a glucose receptor in α- and β-pancreatic cells (Gerich et al., 1973). The work of Goldstein and his group during the last two years has shown that familial hypercholesterolemia, which is transmitted as an autosomal dominant trait is due to a receptor defect of low density lipoproteins (Goldstein and Brown, 1974).

It is our opinion that in the near future in the above mentioned defects as well as in other clinically already well defined conditions hormone receptor defects might be identified as the basis of the disease. Thus, besides chromosomal anomalies and inborn errors of metabolism, hormone receptor defects represent a third class of genetically defined defects, resulting in disturbances of development.

REFERENCES

Attardi, B., and S. Ohno: Cytosol androgen receptor from kidney of normal and testicular feminized (Tfm) mice. Cell 2, 205–212 (1974)

Ballard, P.L., and R.A. Ballard: Glucocorticoid receptors and the role of glucocorticoids in fetal lung development. Proc. Nat. Acad. Sci. (USA) *69*, 2668–2672 (1972)

Bardin, C.W., G.T. Ross, A.B. Rifkind, C.M. Cargille, and M.B. Lipsett: Studies of the pituitary-Leydig cell axis in young men with hypogonadotropic hypogonadism and hyposmia: Comparison with normal men, prepuberal boys and hypopituitary patients. J. Clin. Invest. *48*, 2046–2056 (1969)

Bell, N.H., S. Avery, T. Sinha, C.M. Clark, D.O. Allen, and C. Johnston: Effects of dibutyryl cyclic adenosine 3', 5'-monophosphate and parathyroid extract on calcium and phosphorus metabolism in hypoparathyroidism and pseudohypoparathyroidism. J. Clin Invest. 51, 816–823 (1972)

Boczkowski, K.: Testicular feminization syndrome wihout and with sexual hair. Obstetrics and Gynecology *38*, 719–723 (1971)

Bonati, B., P. Marrama, and L. Della Casa: The "Fertile Eunuch" syndrome: Primary or hypogonadotrophic dissociated hypogonadism? In: The endocrine function of the human testis, Vol. II. V.H.T. James, M. Serio, and L. Martini (eds.). Academic Press, New York and London, pp. 161–180 (1974)

Chase, L.R., G.L. Melson, and G.D. Aurbach: Pseudohypoparathyroidism: Defective excretion of 3', 5'-AMP in response to parathyroid hormone. J. Clin. Invest. *48*, 1832–1844 (1969)

Del Pozo, E.: Pseudohypogonadism: Defective masculinization in a subject with normal FSH, ICSH and testosterone secretion. Horm. Metab. Res. 4, 388–391 (1972)

Fambrough, D.M., D.B. Drachman, and S. Satyamurti: Neuromuscular junction in myasthenia gravis: decreased acetylcholine receptors. Science *182*, 293–295 (1973)

Fichman, M.P., and G. Brooker: Deficient renal cyclic adenosine 3',5'-monophosphate production in nephrogenic diabetes insipidus. J. Clin. Endocrinol. Metab. *35*, 35–47 (1972)

Gehring, U., and G.M. Tomkins: A new mechanism for steroid unresponsiveness: Loss of nuclear binding activity of a steroid hormone receptor. Cell *3*, 301–306 (1974)

Gehring, U., and G.M. Tomkins: Characterization of a hormone receptor defect in the androgen-insensitivity mutant. Cell *3*, 59–64 (1974)

Gerich, J.E., M. Langlois, C. Noacco, J.H. Karam, and P.H. Forsman: Lack of glucagon response to hypoglycemia in diabetes: evidence for an intrinsic pancreatic alpha cell defect. Science *182*, 171–173 (1973)

Goebert, H.W.: Hoch klingt das Lied vom deutschen Gartenzwerg. Badische Zeitung, Oktober 26/27, (1974)

Goldstein, J.L., and M.S. Brown: Binding and degradation of low density lipoproteins by cultured human fibroblasts. J. Biol. Chem. *249*, 5153–5162 (1974)

Keenan, B.S., W.J. Meyer, A.J. Hadjian, H.W. Jones, and C.J. Migeon: Syndrome of androgen insensitivity in man: Absence of 5α-dihydrotesterone binding protein in skin fibroblasts. J. Clin. Endocrinol. Metab. *38*, 1143–1146 (1974)

Kelch, R., S.L. Kaplan, E.G. Biglieri, G.H. Daniels, C.J. Epstein, and M.M. Grumbach: Hereditary adrenocortical unresponsiveness to adrenocorticotropic hormone. J. Pediatr. *81*, 726–736 (1972)

Kim, M.H.: "Gonadotropin-resistant ovaries" syndrome in association with secondary amenorrhea. Am. J. Obstet. Gynecol. *120*, 257–263 (1974)

Kupperman, H.S.: Human endocrinology. Philadelphia, 1963

Lyon, M.F., and S.G. Hawkes: An X-linked gene for testicular feminization of the mouse. Nature *227*, 1217–1219 (1970)

Meyer, W.J., B.R. Migeon, and C.J. Migeon: Locus on human X-chromosome for dihydrotestosterone receptor and androgen insensitivity. Proc. Nat. Acad. Sci. (USA) *72*, 1469–1472 (1975)

Milin, B., and A.K. Roy: Androgen "receptor" in rat liver: Cytosol "receptor" defiency in pseudohermaphrodite male rats. Nature New Biol. (London) *242*, 248–250 (1973)

Ohno, S.: Molecular biology of sex differentiation. Hereditas *69*, 107–124 (1971)

Ohno, S.: Ancient linkage groups and frozen accidents. Nature (London) *244*, 259–262 (1973)

Ohno, S.: Animal model: X-linked testicular feminization mutation of the mouse. Amer. J. Path. *76*, 589–592 (1974)

Quiring, H.: Geschichte des Goldes. Enke, Stuttgart, 1948

Refetoff, S., L.T. DeWind, and L.J. DeGroot: Familial syndrome combining deaf-mutism, stippled epiphyses, goiter and abnormally high PBI: Possible target organ refractoriness to thyroid hormone. J. Clin. Endocr. *27*, 279–294 (1967)

Rimoin, D.L., T.J. Merimee, D. Rabinowitz, V.A. McKusick, and L.L. Cavalli-Sforza: Growth hormone in African pygmies. Lancet *2*, 523–526 (1967)

Rimoin, D.L., T.J. Merimee, D. Rabinowitz, L.L. Cavalli-Sforza, and V.A. McKusick: Peripheral subresponsiveness to human growth hormone in the african pygmies. New Engl. J. Med. *281*, 1383–1388 (1969)

Schultz, P., and D. R. Lines: Nephrogenic diabetes insipidus in an Australian aboriginal kindred. Humangenetik *26*, 79–85 (1975)

Short, R.V.: Reproduction. Ann. Rev. Physiol. *29*, 373–400 (1967)

Sibley, C.H., and G.M. Tomkins: Mechanisms of steroid resistance. Cell *2*, 221–227 (1974)

Stanbury, J.B., P. Rocmans, U.K. Buhler, and Y. Ochi: Congenital hypothyroidism with impaired thyroid response to thyrotropin. New Engl. J. Med. *21*, 1132–1136 (1968)

Wilkins, L.: The diagnosis and treatment of endocrine disorders in childhood and adolescence. Charles C. Thomas, Springfield, III. (1965)

CHROMOSOMAL AND DNA DAMAGE IN PERIPHERAL BLOOD LYMPHOCYTES OF INDIVIDUALS EXPOSED TO KNOWN OR SUSPECTED MUTAGENS: PROBLEMS AND PERSPECTIVES

H. J. EVANS

The availability of simple and efficient techniques for obtaining preparations of human chromosomes from short term cultures of peripheral blood lymphocytes, have enabled man's chromosomes to be studied at the population level. Early studies confirmed that human lymphocyte chromosomes respond to mutagens in the same way as chromosomes of other species, and that the degree of chromosome damage ("chromosome mutation") was directly related to the level of exposure. It is generally accepted that environmental conditions that result in such chromosome damage in somatic cells, produce similar effects in germ cells and germ cell precursors, and there is some evidence from man, and a great deal of evidence from other species, to support this premise. Analyses of mutational changes in human blood lymphocyte nuclei are, therefore, of value for two reasons: (1) they provide us with some direct information on somatic mutation induced in the exposed individual, and in this way should be able to provide us with a useful population monitoring system, and (2) they provide indirect information on possible germ cell mutation.

For the cytogeneticist examining blood cells from exposed individuals, there would appear to be four possible end-points which could yield information on the degree of exposure. These are: (1) the incidence of cells containing more or less than the normal diploid chromosome number; (2) the frequency of chromosomes which are grossly altered in structure as a consequence of breakage and exchange (aberration frequency); (3) the induction of a DNA synthesis outside the normal replication phase of the cell cycle (unscheduled DNA synthesis); and (4) changes in chromosome substructure expressed as sister chromatid exchanges (SCE). For any one of these four systems to be of use in monitoring population exposure to mutagens, it must meet with a number of requirements the four most important being: (1) that the system is stable with a low background or noise level; (2) that it is highly sensitive to mutagen exposure; (3) that changes in the degree of damage detected by the system must bear a strict quantitative relationship to the level of exposure; and (4) that any alterations in the system must be such that they may be detected over a considerable period of time after exposure.

1. *Alterations in chromosome number*

Exposure of cells to mutagens frequently results in a loss of one or more chromosomes at an ensuing cell division. It might be expected, therefore, that the presence of a significant proportion of hypodiploid cells might well reflect a previous mutagenic exposure. A major problem here, however, is the high and somewhat variable background level. Our studies in Edingburgh on populations that have not been unduly exposed to known mutagens, show us that the incidence of hypodiploidy in peripheral blood lymphocytes is somewhere around 1 or 2 % in young individuals, and that this incidence increases up to around 10 % in ageing members of the population. The marked increase associated with age is due to a loss of the inactive X chromosome from cells in the female and of the Y chromosome in cells from the male. Thus, although one might expect to be able to detect increased hypodiploidy in individuals exposed to high doses of mutagen, the background, or noise, level is rather high and the system would appear to be too insensitive to be used for population monitoring.

2. *Gross changes in chromosome structure*

Changes in chromosome structure involve breakages and exchange of chromosome parts and they are basically of two sorts: *chromatid-type* aberrations in which the unit of breakage and exchange is the single chromatid or half-chromosome, and *chromosome-type* aberrations in which the unit of breakage is a whole chromosome, both chromatids being involved at identical loci in any breakage or exchange process. Chromatid changes represent breaks and exchanges that occur at or following the replication of chromosomes in interphase, whereas chromosome aberrations are formed at early interphase prior to replication. The distinction between these two types of aberration is important since some mutagens, for example ionizing radiations, produce only chromosome-type changes in exposed blood lymphocytes, whereas others produce lesions that develop into aberrations when the cells proceed through a DNA replication phase, so that the aberrations produced are exclusively of the chromatid-type.

In the case of chromatid-type aberrations, studies on many thousands of cells scored from many hundreds of individuals in work carried out at our laboratory show that less than 0.5 % of blood lymphocytes show chromatid deletions and that the incidence of chromatid interchanges is probably less than one in every 4,000 cells examined. It seems fairly clear, therefore, that, under well-defined conditions, chromatid-type aberrations which involve changes in structure are rather rare events in blood cells from unexposed individuals.

Similar kinds of information are available on chromosome-type aberrations, and here particular emphasis has been paid to the dicentric chromosome-type aberration which is rarely found in cells of unexposed individuals, but is of common occurrence if people have been exposed to ionizing radiations. Again data from many thousands of cells from over 2,000 people have shown that the incidence of dicentric changes is low, and is of the order of around 1 in 4,000 cells. It is clear, therefore, that the background frequency of chromosome aberrations is low.

Insofar as sensitivity of chromosomes to structural changes is concerned, there is ample information now from *in vitro* and *in vivo* studies showing that one can detect effects of X-rays at levels of around 15 rads, where significant numbers of dicentric aberrations are to be found. Much of the data on chromosome damage induced in man by ionizing radiation has come from studies on patients exposed in hospital and from occupationally exposed industrial workers. In addition, there is some information available from individuals exposed accidentally, and from all these data it is evident that not only can we easily detect the effects of quite low doses of X-rays shortly after a person has been exposed, but that the frequency of aberrations declines slowly with time, and indeed in some cases drops to around 50 % of the initial level some three years or so after exposure. It is thus possible to obtain a history of radiation exposure sometime after the population has actually been exposed.

In summary, as far as ionizing radiations are concerned, it is clear that we can detect the chromosome damaging effects of quite low doses at a population level and that these damaging effects may be detectable up to a number of years after the receipt of original exposure.

The information available on chromosome damage induced in individuals exposed to chemical mutagens is in no way as comprehensive as that available on people exposed to ionizing radiations.

Studies have been carried out on groups of individuals exposed to benzene, lead, cadmium, and various other possible mutagens, with some mixed results. There are a variety of problems in interpreting these results, not least being the fact that with many chemical mutagens the aberrations may be made when cells carrying lesions in their DNA are stimulated to proceed through the replication phase. These lesions may be repaired long before a lymphocyte enters a proliferating phase, so that no aberrations will be produced. However, cells that were proliferating in the body at the time of exposure, e.g. epithelial cells and gonad cells, will nevertheless have suffered genetic damage which may pass undetected in samples of blood lymphocytes taken sometime later. Obviously we need more *in vivo* information on the effects of known chemical mutagens, but this work is still at a somewhat preliminary stage.

3. *Unscheduled DNA synthesis*

Peripheral blood lymphocytes are normally in the G_0 or G_1 phase of the cell cycle and do not usally undergo DNA synthesis whilst in the peripheral circulation. However, if they are exposed to mutagens which produce DNA damage, the damage may be repaired by a process of repair replication which involves a measure of DNA synthesis. This "unscheduled" DNA synthesis can be detected if the cells are incubated in the presence of ^{3}H-thymidine, and the incorporation of the labelled precursor measured by autoradiography or scintillation counting. The induction of unscheduled DNA synthesis has been considered to provide a valuable test for mutagenicity and carcinogenicity in *in vitro* systems, and we should consider whether this phenomenon can be used as a monitor for population exposure.

We have studied unscheduled DNA synthesis, *in vitro,* in human lymphocytes exposed to ionizing radiations or to a wide variety of chemical mutagens. Insofar as ionizing radiations are concerned, it is clear that detectable amounts of newly synthesised DNA are only to be found in cells exposed to doses of above about 500 rads – a very high dose level. Similarly, in the case of many chemical mutagens, to obtain any significant incorporation of label the cells have to be subjected to a dose that would result in killing a major fraction of the cell population. It would appear, therefore, that this particular system is rather insensitive, despite the fact that there is very little background or noise. A further difficulty here is that the incorporation of label into newly synthesized DNA is largely completed within a few hours after exposure for the majority of mutagens tested.

In summary then, our data on unscheduled DNA synthesis suggest that this phenomenon will not be a useful marker to monitor exposure of populations to mutagens.

4. Changes in chromosome substructure (sister chromatid exchange)

Recently a number of new techniques have been developed which have enabled us to readily visualize sister chromatid exchanges induced in chromosomes following their exposure to mutagens. These exchange events take place between sister DNA double helices within a chromosome and they probably reflect recombinational repair events. We have now studied the incidence of sister chromatid exchange (SCE) in cells from a variety of individuals and shown that, with extremely rare exceptions, the background frequency is pretty constant between cells and people, with an average incidence of around 12 SCE per cell. If these cells are exposed to ionizing radiations, there is an increase in the frequency of SCE but the doses required to produce significant increases are large, e.g. at about 400 rads there is just over a doubling in the incidence of SCE. This particular end-point, therefore, is unlikely to be value in monitoring populations for exposure to ionizing radiations. On the other hand, the incidence of SCE in cells exposed to certain chemical mutagens is extremely high, even following low-dose exposure. For example, exposure to Mitomycin C at concentrations of around 10^{-8} molar, over two cell cycles, gives a 40-fold increase in SCE frequency. Studies on 20 different chemical mutagens in *in vitro* systems have shown that the majority of these mutagens produce large increases in SCE, and it would seem that this might provide a system for monitoring populations exposed to chemical agents. Preliminary results on patients exposed to a variety of cytotoxic drugs have shown that we can pick up increased SCE frequencies in blood cells in the early days following exposure, and further studies in this area will place us in a better position to assess the promise of this approach for population monitoring.

In conclusion, we can say that lymphocyte chromosome aberrations provide a good system for monitoring population exposure to ionizing radiations. A major problem here is the tedium involved in searching for and analysing the large number of dividing cells that need to be examined to detect low level effects. However, there are a number of significant advances that have been made towards automating the process of cell finding and analysis, and in the very near future it is expected that this kind of monitoring may be carried out by machine. Insofar as chemical mutagens are concerned, we clearly need a lot more information, but, in principal, chromosome aberration incidence might also provide a useful monitoring system for chemical exposures. However, the results indicate that testing for DNA repair by detecting *in vitro* incorporation of labelled DNA precursors post-exposure would seem to have little merit. On the other hand, the detection of DNA lesions that give rise to sister chromatid exchange seems a very promising approach, but further work is necessary here before we can decide if this approach will provide us with a sensitive and useful system to monitor damage in exposed populations.

PRENATAL MONITORING FOR CONGENITAL DISEASES

H. GALJAARD AND M.F. NIERMEIJER

An increasing number of centres in more and more countries have started the service of prenatal diagnosis to parents at risk for those congenital disorders that can be detected by analysis of amniotic fluid (cells). This new tool in genetic counseling is sometimes underestimated and on the other hand its purpose and significance has been exaggerated. Prenatal detection of congenital diseases followed by interruption of the pregnancy in case an affected fetus is found, is not yet a potent means in the prevention of physically and/or mentally handicapped people. At the individual scale however, it offers new perspectives for parents who are at (high) risk for a seriously affected child. Sometimes this concerns parents who already gave birth to one or more abnormal children and as a result of this do not dare a next pregnany; in other instances, like in carriers of X-linked diseases or chromosomal translocations or in women at advanced age the fear of getting an affected child prevents their possibility of extending the family with normal children. The knowledge that in a (next) pregnancy prenatal tests can be performed may eliminate the fear of the parents.

In Table I the main indication groups and the (recurrence) risks involved are listed.

Cromosomal aberrations can be detected by karyotyping cultivated amniotic fluid cells and such studies are usually completed 10–14 days after transabdominal amniocentesis in the 14th – 16th week of pregnancy. In different European centres over 3500 of such prenatal diagnoses have been made mainly in pregnancies where the mother was older than 38 years or in pregnancies where an earlier child with a chromosomal aberration (mostly trisomy 21 in Down's syndrome) had been born. In our own group in Rotterdam out of about 300 pregnancies monitored on a chromosomal aberration 10 affected fetuses were detected (trisomy 21 and 18, 47XXY, 47XYY, unbalanced translocations). In all these instances the parents chose for interruption of the pregnancy. The technique of fetal karyotyping does not give major problems in the hands of experienced groups, and

Table I: Main indications for prenatal diagnosis and risks for a congenital disease

Chromosomal aberrations	
– advanced maternal age (> 38 years)	1– 2 % for Down's syndrome
– previous child with chromosomal aberration	1– 2 % for Down's syndrome
– parental translocation	10–50 % for Down's syndrome
X-linked diseases	
– Hemophilia, Duchenne's muscular dystrophy etc.	50 % affected males if mother is carrier
Metabolic disorders	
– about 50 enzyme deficiencies involved in carbohydrate- lipid-, aminoacid and nucleic acid metabolism	25 % if parents are carrier
Open neural tube defects	
– previous child with anencephaly or open spina bifida	
– one of parents affected	3–5 %

prenatal diagnosis should in my opinion be centralized in these groups. Only if it becomes apparent that the number of requests will exceed the capacity of a certain centre a new group should be trained. The total number of centres required in a country depends on the number of annual births, the proportion of elderly mothers (in Holland about 2,5 % over 40 years) and the percentage of couples that want prenatal tests to be performed. Unfortunately, about this last aspect little is known about the different factors that result in the discrepancy between the number of mothers at risk and those who undergo prenatal monitoring.

Sex-linked diseases will be transmitted by a carrier mother to 50 % of her sons. For some of these diseases the basic biochemical defect is known like the muco-polysaccharidosis II (Hunter's disease), lipidosis of Fabry and the Lesch-Nyhan syndrome. In these instances it can be demonstrated whether or not a male fetus is affected. However, there are over 150 X-linked disorders for which the biochemical defect has not yet been classified. Two of the most frequent examples of such diseases are progressive muscular dystrophy type Duchenne and hemophilia A. In pregnancies at risk for these or other serious X-linked diseases the fetal sex can be determined and in case a female fetus is found the parents can be reassured; and if a male fetus is detected the parents may want interruption of their pregnancy thus preventing the birth of an (other) affected son. A problem in this type of prenatal monitoring is that in case of a male fetus there is a 50 % chance that this is unaffected. Notwithstanding this disadvantage many hundreds of parents at risk for X-linked disease have asked for prenatal sex determination in order to be able to extend their family with healthy daughters without the risk of an affected son. In our own group we have performed about 50 such analyses and as expected half of these revealed male sex. Prenatal sex determination should always be based on the investigation of a complete fetal karyotype; so far all predicted fetal sexes proved to be correct.

Inborn errors of metabolism can also be detected in early pregnancy in case the basic biochemical defect is known and can be demonstrated in cultured fluid cells. At present this is the case for about 50 metabolic diseases more than 90 % of which are of autosomal recessive inheritance. This means that in nearly all instances it will be detected that both parents are carrier of the same gene mutation after that the diagnosis of their first affected child has been established. Prenatal diagnosis can then only contribute to the prevention of the birth of a following handicapped child in the same family for which otherwise a 25 % risk exists. In the case of the few X-linked diseases it might be known that a woman is carrier before she has her first pregnancy. This will be so if she has affected brothers and/or uncles and also biochemical tests can be performed to establish the carriership. Subsequently prenatal monitoring can already be performed in the first pregnancy and hence the birth of the first affected child can be prevented.

Each of the inborn errors of metabolism occurs rather infrequently and so far not more than a few hundred prenatal diagnoses have been established for about 20 metabolic diseases. If cell cultivation, harvesting and biochemical analyses are performed properly and using the right control material prenatal diagnosis has shown to be reliable; this is not the case if enzyme analyses are performed on amniotic fluid supernatant!

When conventional biochemical assay procedures are used it mostly took 4,5 weeks to collect sufficient cell material for an enzyme assay. In case storage of specific metabolites has to be demonstrated (like cystinosis or mucopolysaccharidoses) generally, more cell material and hence longer waiting periods are required. By using small (0.1–1 μl) incubation volumes and measuring the resulting fluorescence or extinction in microcuvettes (10–50 μl) the sensivity of the enzyme analyses can be improved and the cultivation period can be reduced to about 2 weeks. If special preparation techniques are used, enabling the isolation of small groups (10th–100^{ds}) of cultured amniotic fluid cells, and measurements are performed in glass-capillaries using a microscope spectrofluorometer the prenatal diagnosis of certain metabolic diseases can even be established 7–10 days after amniocentesis. In our own group about 40 prenatal diagnoses of 12 different inborn errors of metabolism have been established. For most of these, microchemical techniques were used enabling a diagnosis of the tests within 7–18 days after amniocentesis. For a reliable diagnosis it is essential that the analytical data are compared with those of primary cultures of control amniotic fluid cells grown under identical conditions.

Congenital malformations as a result of disturbances during embryonic development are generally not amenable for prenatal diagnosis except open neural tube defects such as spina bifida and anencephaly. If the fetus is affected with one of these diseases the content of α-foetoprotein in the amniotic fluid supernatant is markedly increased around the 16th week of pregnancy.

The main problems in prenatal diagnosis are no longer of a technical nature provided that the amniocenteses (or under ultrasound control) by an experienced subsequent cell cultivation and chromosomal or biochemical analyses are carried out by groups that have sufficient experience. The most important problem to be solved is to detect in time which parents are at risk for an affected child and to organize the screening, diagnosis and genetic counseling in such a way that the parents concerned can make use of prenatal monitoring when this is indicated.

GENETIC HETEROGENEITY IN METABOLIC DISORDER STUDIED BY SOMATIC CELL HYBRIDIZATION

H. GALJAARD and A. J. J. REUSER

At present in about 10 % of the 2000 monogenic congenital diseases the basic biochemical defect has been clarified. This enables an exact diagnosis by performing enzyme analysis of organ biopsies, blood (cells) or cultured skin fibroblasts; for those diseases where the enzymic defect is detectable in cultured amniotic fluid cells prenatal monitoring can be carried out thus enabling prevention of the disease concerned.

For an increasing number of metabolic disorders it becomes clear that there are different clinical and/or biochemical variants. In patients with the same clinical symptoms the residual activity or the properties of the deficient enzyme may differ. Also "the same" enzyme deficiency is sometimes resulting in different clinical and pathological manifestations. For many metabolic disorders infantile, juvenile and adult forms have now been described but in most cases the underlying mechanisms are not yet clear. Further insight in the relation between gene mutation, enzyme deficiency, pathological and clinical abnormalities can be gained by somatic cell hybridization studies and investigation of the properties and functions of the (deficient) enzyme. In this paper a few examples of such studies are presented with the aim of elucidating the genetic background of different variants of some lysosomal storage diseases.

Like in unicellular organisms, enzyme deficient human cells can be hybridized and genetic complementation, i.e. restoration of enzyme activity not present in both parental cell strains, indicates that two different gene mutations are responsible for the enzyme deficiency concerned. Bootsma's group [1] has for the first time showed such complementation to occur after fusion of skin fibroblasts derived from two patients with different variants of an inherited disturbance in nucleic acid metabolism. Later on Barbara Migeon's group [2] and our own group [3] independently showed that the Tay-Sachs and the Sandhoff variant of GM2 gangliosidosis are based on two different gene mutations. These conclusions were reached by hybridization of about 10^6 cultured fibroblasts from each patient, a few days of subsequent cultivation and enzymatic analysis of the hybridized cell proliferation; whereas hexosaminidase A activity lacked in both parental cell strains it could clearly been demonstrated as soon as 24–48 hours after fusion of both cell strains.

More recently our group has been able to genetically classify 4 different clinical variants of GM1 gangliosidosis; although the pathological and clinical manifestations varied markedly among the different patients a profound β-galactosidase deficiency was present in cells from all patients. Enzyme analyses both with artificial and natural substrate (the latter being carried out by Mae Wan Ho, Dept. Biochemistry Queen Elizabeth College, London) at two days after hybridization of fibroblasts from the various patients showed two complementation groups. The types 1 and 2 MG1 gangliosidosis [4] are caused by different gene mutations than Pinsky's type [5] 3 and the adult type 4 described by our own group [6]. So far we were not able to detect any genetic differences between type 1 and 2 or between type 3 and 4.

By using microchemical methods enabling enzyme assays on single cultured (hybrid) cells we could demonstrate that in at least one type of fusion (types 1 x 4) the genetic complementation results in a restoration of β-galactosidase activity comparable to that in control fibroblasts.

Complementation analyses of cells from a patient with an early diagnosed enzyme deficiency with cells from patients with already known clinical course will not only result in an exact genetic classification but may also give information about the clinical prognosis.

We have performed several other hybridization experiments involving infantile and adult types of glycogenosis II (α – 1.4 glucosidase deficiency), different types of G6PD deficiency and different clinical and biochemical variants of metachromatic leucodystrophy and mucolipidosis where arylsulfatase isoenzymes are deficient. In more of these fusion combinations we have so far observed genetic complementation. This shows that not all different biochemical and clinical variants can be traced back to different gene mutations. So far there is no evidence that allelic mutations result in genetic complementation since Nadler's suggestion of intraallelic complementation after fusion of different variants of galactosemia has never been confirmed. In those cases where hitherto genetic complementation has clearly been demonstrated the exact molecular structure of the enzymes involved or the precise nature of the enzymic deficiency has not yet been resolved; it is therefore still possible that what is now believed to be interallelic complementation is in fact the result of deficiencies in different enzymes and/or other regulator substances. Further studies involving cell hybridization, biochemical and immunological investigations of the properties of the (deficient) enzyme are likely to provide important information not only about the background of different clinical variants of metabolic disorders but also on the molecular genetics and cellular biochemistry of the proteins involved.

REFERENCES

[1] Weerd-Kastelein, E.A., de, Keijzer, W. and Bootsma, D., Nature *238*, 80 (1972)

[2] Thomas, G.H., Taylor, H.A., Miller, C.S., Axelman, J. and Migeon, B.R., Nature, *250*, 580 (1974)

[3] Galjaard, H., Hoogeveen, A., Wit-Verbeek, H.A. de, Reuser, A.J.J., Kleijer, W., Westerveld, A. and Bootsma, D., Exptl. Cell Res. *87*, 444 (1974)

[4] O'Brien, J.S. in: Advances in Human Genetics, Harris H. and Hirschhorn, K. (eds.) Vol. 3 pp. 39–98, Plenum Press, N.York (1972)

[5] Pinsky, L., Miller, J., Stanfield, B., Watters, G. and Wolfe, L.S., Amer. J. Hum. Genet., *26*, 563 (1974)

[6] Loonen, M.C.B., Lugt, L. v.d. and Franke, C.L., Lancet ii, 785 (1974)

IMMUNE RESPONSE GENES

EBERHARD GÜNTHER

The structure of antibodies (immunoglobulins) which are the most important antigen-specific receptor and effector molecules in the immune response is controlled by three genetically unlinked clusters of genes (i.e. genes for heavy chains, lambda and kappa light chains). The diversity of the antigen combining sites of antibodies resides in the diversity of the v gene set in each of these clusters.

In recent years a group of genes has been described which control immune responsiveness in an antigen-specific manner yet are genetically not linked to the immunoglobulin structural genes, but are linked to the major histocompatibility gene complex. These genes have been termed histocompatibility-linked immune response genes (Ir genes) and have been identified in all higher vertebrates so far tested. Ir genes determine high and low responsiveness, respectively, to a great variety of synthetic and natural antigens, among them potentially pathogenic antigens.

Data on genetic complementation of histocompatibility-linked Ir genes controlling immune responsiveness to certain antigens demonstrate genetic heterogeneity of low responder phenotypes and show that two or more histocompatibility-linked Ir genes are involved in determining high responsiveness to these antigens.

The degree of diversity of Ir genes with respect to antigen specificity is not yet known, neither the mode of generating this diversity nor its relationship to antibody diversity. Therefore, and since in the latter case somatic mutations are discussed as playing a major role in generating diversity and specificity, Ir genes are – at least at present – not useful for mutation monitoring of populations.

TESTING FOR POINT MUTATIONS BY PROTEIN MAPPING

JOACHIM KLOSE

Test systems used to detect induced point mutations in mammals or man make it necessary to examine a large number of samples or animals. There are two possibilities which might be used in order to reduce this large magnitude of work: one is to simplify the technique used for mutagenicity testing. The other possibility is to employ a method which is able to control a higher number of genes. It was already emphasized by Dr. Neel that the electrophoresis of a number of distinct enzymes or other proteins is one of the best means to detect point mutations. On the basis of such a system I further developed a method (Klose, 1975) which allows a large number of proteins to be controlled and which is relatively simple to perform.

Protein mapping method

Applying this method protein samples are separated by migration into two dimensions: the first dimension is effected by isoelectric focusing (pH 3,5–10,0) and the second by electrophoresis. Separation using the first step depends on the isoelectric point of the proteins, separation employing the second step depends on the molecular size of the protein. Different characteristics of the protein molecule are utilized at each given time step and in this way a high resolution is achieved.

The protein sample which we use is a complex protein solution extracted from mouse organs. We extract the cytoplasmatic proteins from the tissue, while at the same time trying to separate the proteins which are bound to the structures of the cells. After the two dimensional separation of the proteins in polyacrylamide gels the protein spots are stained unspecifically with Comassie Blue.

Using this method we are able to detect several hundreds of protein spots from one sample. For example, more than 300 spots are to be obtained from mouse liver. Protein patterns resulting from parallel runs are completely reproducible.

The focusing run is performed within a 5 hr., the second run within a 1 1/2 hr. time period. Presently we have started experiments using an apparatus which was recommended by Dale and Latner (1969). The use of this apparatus allows one to put several gel rods after isoelectric focusing on large slab gels. In this way 8 or 16 samples can be separated at the same time.

When one compares the protein mapping method with a mutagenicity test system, using several enzymes and electrophoretic systems, it is found that the advantage of the protein mapping method lies in the large number of proteins which can be investigated by using only one sample of an individual, one electrophoretic system and one staining solution. Our method may have the disadvantage, that the genetic, biochemistry and function of the proteins utilized are unknown. However, this method is designed as a mutagenicity test for routine investigations. What we are trying to find out is: does one group of animals exposed to a mutagen show more variations in their protein patterns than the control group? Should it arise that we do find a variant protein spot, this protein would then be investigated more closely in detail.

We have modified the protein mapping technique in some ways. The use of Sodium Dodecyl Sulfate (SDS) in the second dimension results in a better distribution of the spots over the gel, and the number of spots is further increased. On the other hand, the use of SDS is responsible for the method being less sensitive to protein charge differences. Furthermore, we have adapted the protein mapping method to investigations on a micro scale. Using this micro method embryos in their early stages can be examined and the possibility exists that mutations can be detected which are lethal in a later stage of embryonic development.

An evaluation of the protein patterns follows by visually examining and comparing the gels. However, we are also trying to evaluate the pattern by the use of a densitometer which is used in collaboration with a computer and a typewriter. To some extent success was achieved with the use of the Quantimet (Imanco GmbH, 605 Offenbach). Employing this apparatus each spot is expressed as a number which reflects the staining intensity of the protein and the numbers are registered two dimensionally according to the protein pattern.

One cannot assume that the number of spots which are visible on the two dimensional protein pattern is identical with the number of genes included within this test system. On the one hand, the number of genes may be higher because several spots may consist of two or three proteins, and variants from each of these proteins should be visible. On the other hand, several spots may be the result of non-genetic processes.

We tried to calculate the number of samples necessary in order to find one spontaneous mutation in mice. For this purpose I shall assume that the protein pattern reflects 250 genes. The mutation rate for electrophoretically detectable spontaneous mutations in man was recently calculated by Dr. Neel (1974) and the result of this was the number $3x10^{-5}$. Applying this number to mice and assuming that the protein pattern reflects 250 genes would mean that 120 samples (animals) would have to be investigated in order to ascertain one spontaneous mutation. Of course, after the animals have been treated with a mutagenic substance, two or more variant protein spots should be detectable within 120 protein patterns. Using this method 120 samples can be easily investigated by one technician within a 2 week time period.

Mapping of proteins from different strains of mice

Employing the protein mapping method we investigated different strains of mice in order to show with the aid of a model that the method used is capable of demonstrating genetically determined variant proteins. A large number of variant protein spots were found. Some of our preliminary results are shown in Table 1. The total number of variants varies from one strain to another. In consideration of these differences it was found that a great genetic distance exists from the strain C57BL/6J to the other three strains investigated. The same finding was made by Taylor (1972), who investigated isoenzymes from different strains of mice by employing conventional electrophoresis. In order to show precisely that the variant proteins found are genetically determined, we investigated hybrids of different strains of mice using the mapping method. Heterozygote patterns were clearly visible for most variants.

Investigation of mice treated with a mutagenic substance (MNU)

Male mice were treated with Methyl-Nitroso-Urea (MNU) and mated with the females at that time when treated Spermatogonia appear in the ejaculat. On day 18 p.c. the liver proteins from single F_1-fetuses were examined using the protein mapping method. We have just initiated this type of experiment in our laboratory and up to now 100 samples (fetal livers) from the treated group and 100 samples from a control group of mice have been investigated. Two variant proteins were found in the treated group and none in the control group. Further experiments will be necessary in order to demonstrate a possible significant effect of MNU and to exclude the possibility of the existence of a certain background variation within an inbred strain of mice. Moreover, experiments will have to be performed in such a way as to allow P-and F_2 generations to be investigated in the case where a mutation is found in a mouse of the F_1 generation.

Table 1: The nomenclature of the variant proteins was chosen arbitrarily in order to characterize them in some respect

Genetically variant liver proteins of four strains of mice														
Strains of mice	Variant protein spots each present only in one strain													Total number
BALB/c Han.	Q^{ap}													1
AKR/J	C^{ap}	C^{m}	F^{ap}	G^{ap}	J^{ap}									5
DBA/2J	T^{ap}	U^{ap}	V^{ap}	G^{m}	F^{i}	H^{m}								6
C57BL/6J	A^{ap}	B^{i}	B^{m}	A^{mix}	D^{ap}	E^{ap}	K^{ap}	L^{ap}	E^{m}	M^{ap}	O^{ap}	P^{ap}	C^{mix}	13
														25
	Variant protein spots each present in two strains													Total number
AKR/J	C^{i}	D^{i}	B^{mix}	R^{ap}	S^{ap}	F^{m}								
C57BL/6J	C^{i}	D^{i}	$B^{mix'}$	R^{ap}	S^{ap}	F^{m}	B^{ap}	D^{m}	H^{ap}	I^{ap}	N^{ap}	A^{i}	$A^{m/i}$	6
BALB/c Han.							B^{ap}	D^{m}	H^{ap}	I^{ap}	N^{ap}			5
DBA/2J												A^{i}	$A^{m/i'}$	2
														13

Mapping of different types of proteins

The protein mapping technique is probably not very useful as a method for monitoring human populations (using serum, for example), since one can expect that such complex protein patterns differ from one individual to another in a wild population. However, one can assume that certain protein types display no natural polymorphisms. In this instance one could restrict this method to proteins of this type.

In respect to problems of population monitoring the protein mapping method could be useful for another reason. The method allows variant proteins in complex protein solutions to be detected, for example, in the cytoplasm of a certain tissue. Therefore, the method offers the possibility of probing for genetic variability in quite different types of proteins, each including a large number of single proteins. Possible protein types which could be investigated are the following: cytoplasmatic proteins, membrane proteins, chromosomal proteins, ribosomal proteins; proteins specific to certain tissues or developmental stages; proteins which differ markedly in molecular weight or amino acid composition. The main question to be answered is whether one can find a few proteins or a group of proteins which show much more frequent mutations than other proteins. Such proteins (if they can be easily won from man) could be used further as an indicator within an electrophoretic system for population monitoring. Their use would reduce the large number of individuals actually necessary for a monitoring program. There could be several reasons for the appearance of mutations with different frequencies in different proteins. For example: gaps in the proteins covering the DNA would make it possible that a mutagen acts more intensively at certain DNA sequences. The mutation of a gene which occurs repeatedly would never be detectable at the protein level. Another possibility could be that a substitution of an amino acid in certain proteins results more often in an electrophoretic variant protein, which is due to the higher content of charged amino acids in this protein. The investigation of different types of proteins under the aspect as to which proteins undergo mutations at the highest frequency should be done on the basis of investigating new-mutations, for example, by investigating closely related sublines of mice or, if possible, by investigating induced point mutations. Investigations aimed at detecting proteins of different degrees of variability could be much more easily accomplished on the basis of investigating balanced polymorphisms. However, if two different groups of proteins are found, the difference could stem predominantly from the natural selection and the genetic drift and not from the mutation process itself.

Regarding the balanced polymorphisms it is interesting to know that two different groups of proteins were found. Harris et al. (1974) have shown that enzymes can be divided into polymorphic and monomorphic proteins. Gillespie et al. (1968) formulated the hypothesis that the degree of polyporphism is related to the function of the enzymes. Johnson (1973) described two groups of enzymes. One group, which utilizes external substrates, shows a higher level of genetic variability than the other group, which utilizes internal metabolites. Applying the protein mapping technique we investigated proteins from different mouse organs and compared the protein patterns of different strains. Some of the preliminary results are shown in Table 2. Certain organs show relatively more variant proteins than other organs. When the total number of spots found for each organ is categorically divided into spots present in several organs and spots seen only in one organ

Table 2: Protein spots of C57BL/6J-mice in comparison with the protein spots of AKR/J-mice

Organs	Spots of organs			Spots common to several organs	Organ "specific" spots
	total number of spots	number of variant spots (mutations)	variant spots / total number of spots %	variant spots / total number of spots %	variant spots / total number of spots %
liver	325	26	8,00	5,75	11,11
kidney	305	20	6,56	5,36	10,63
brain	290	10	3,45	4,37	1,60
muscle	188	5	2,66	4,08	0,00
serum	148	4	2,70		

("specific" spots), it is obvious that the organs will differ markedly in the frequency of variants found in the groups of "specific" proteins. Therefore, proteins, for instance, "specific" to the brain, proteins "specific" to the liver or proteins common to several organs may represent three different types of proteins, which differ in function, structure or/and genes. This may account for the different levels of genetic variability present in these types of proteins.

In conclusion, two staetments can be made. 1) The protein mapping method seems to be applicable to a test system which is used to detect induced point mutations in mammals. This method is efficacious because only one electrophoretic system is needed in order to survey a large number of proteins. 2) The protein mapping method makes the detection possible of proteins which show mutations at a high frequency. Such proteins would be especially suitable for a monitoring system because the number of individuals necessary for a monitoring program can be reduced in this way.

REFERENCES

Klose, J., Humangenetik 26, 231 (1975)

Dale, G., Latner, A.L., Clin. Chim. Acta 24, 61 (1969)

Neel, J.V., Mutation Res. 26, 319 (1974)

Taylor, B.A., J. Heredity 63, 83 (1972)

Harris, H., Hopkinson, D.A., Robson, E.B., Ann. Hum. Genet., Lond. 37, 237 (1974)

Gillespie, J., Kojima, K., Proc. Nat. Acad. Sci. US 6, 582 (1968)

Johnson, G., Nature New Biology 243, 151 (1973)

POSSIBLE ADVANTAGES AND DISADVANTAGES OF NON-TRANSMITTED, SINGLE-CELL HUMAN MUTAGENESIS ASSAYS

CHARLES H. LANGLEY and KENNY CRUMP

It is quite natural to seek relevant human mutation assays from readily available cells. Professor Evans has discussed the present situation as far as cytogenetic endpoints are concerned. The other major possibility is the biochemical one. Because of the work in this area at Niehs, we have considered some advantages and disadvantages that are likely to be associated with the utilization of such non-transmitted, single-cell mutagenic assays.

The most readily available cells are, of course, blood cells and perhaps sperm. The quantification of stem cell dynamics in spermatogenesis is significantly better than that for hemopoiesis although for most of the following discussion, they are qualitatively similar. So we construct a simple model of the population dynamics of spermatogenesis and investigate its sampling properties. Consider a single cell (fertilized ova) that divides until at puberty there are some 10^7–10^8 stem cells in the mature male gonad. Assuming a particular mutation is selectively neutral, the expected frequency of mutant stem cells at puberty is $E(q) = \mu 1nN$ where μ is the per cell generation mutation rate and N is the number of stem cells at maturity (Luria and Delbrück) [1]. The variance of this frequency is $Var(q) = \mu$. Consider now that after puberty, these stem cells undergo simple linear replacement. The expected frequency of mutants after n post-puberty generations is $E(q) = \mu_0 LnN + n\mu_1$ where μ_1 is the post-puberty per cell generation rate and the variance is for these practical purposes still $Var(q) = \mu_0$. Since the determinaton of mutant frequencies in the cells of particular individuals at particular times will be highly automated, we will assume no sampling error at this level. Note again that we are considering hypothetical phenotypes that are selectively neutral. Now let us examine several possible situations where such a scheme might be applied.

In the following cases, we have resorted to normal approximations which are adequate for indication of sample size effects.

Case 1. A group of factory workers are being exposed to a suspected mutagen. We assume that the normal spontaneous rate is known and that the factory workers had this known pre-puberty mutation rate of $\mu_o = 10^{-6}$. Post-puberty, the normal population also has a per cell generation mutation rate of $10^{-6} = \mu_o$ and the factory workers μ_f. Thus we are testing the factory workers against a „known“ normal rate. How large a sample of factory workers would be needed to detect the increase μ_f/μ_o? From Table 1, we see that large numbers would be needed to detect even large effects.

Table 1: Sample sizes needed to detect the increase in mutation rate $\mu_f > \mu_o$
$\mu_o = 10^{-6}$ (known)
$\alpha = 0.05/\ \beta = 0.1/$ one tailed.

μ_f/μ_o	Years of Post-puberty Exposure					
	0.1	0.5	1	5	10	20
2		124600	31200	1245	311	78
10	38500	1538	385	15	4	

Case 2. Suppose two populations are exposed lifelong to different concentrations of some agents. That is, one population has a pre- and post-puberty rate of $10^{-6} = \mu_1$ and the other a larger rate of μ_2. Samples of equal size are drawn from each population.

Table 2: Sample size (K) needed to detect the increase in mutation rate $\mu_2 > \mu_1$ (both unknown). $\mu_o = 10^{-6}$,
$\alpha_o = 0.05/\ \beta = 0.1/$ one tailed.

μ_2/μ_1	Years of Post-puberty Exposure		
	0	5	20
1.5	555041	8717	664
2	155460	3191	186

From Table 2, we find that the sample sizes needed from each population are indeed big, too late and only after large exposures.

Despite these pessimistic tables, we can identify several technical developments that may still leave the non-transmitted single-cell mutagenesis assay with much utility. The first and most obvious is the simultaneous assay of more than one phenotypic class. If the number of loci being assayed per individual is ten rather than one, then the sample sizes needed are one-tenth of those in the tables.

The second and more important technical development that we have not included in our model today is a serial sampling scheme. By doing this, the large variance among individuals would play no role and small changes might be more easily detected. The utility of a serial sampling scheme will hinge to a large extent on the variability in the dynamics of a stem cell population. If this is large, then the utility will be diminished.

Despite the sense of caution, we must recognize that nontransmitted single cell mutation assays offer the only possible assay of mutagenic insult in the practical epidemiology situation. If we have to wait a whole generation to detect an effect via transmitted endpoints, the damage will have been done.

REFERENCE

[1] Luria, S. E., and Delbrück, M., Mutations of bacteria from virus sensitivity to virus resistance. Genetics *28*: 491–511, 1943.

ADVANTAGES AND DISADVANTAGES OF HISTOCOMPATIBILITY GENES IN MONITORING THE TREND OF THE MUTATION RATE

ALENA LENGEROVÁ

The polymorphism of histocompatibility genes (briefly H-genes) is responsible for antigenic uniqueness of the individual which is reflected in the fact that cells, tissues or organs of one individual (the donor) transplanted to another individual (the recipient) are recognized by the immune system of the latter as "non-self" and are rejected. For several reasons, H-genes could well be considered as candidates for monitoring a possible trend of the mutation rate in the human population. Their potential advantages may be listed as follows.

1) Among numerous H-genes in mammalian species, one presents the main obstacle to successful tissue transplantation. There is thus an understandable tendency to avoid incompatibility at this so-called "major H-gene complex" (which is the HL-A system in man) by matching the donor and recipient of organ transplants for antigens of this particular system. On the basis of antigenic polymorphism, HL-A variants can be detected relatively easily by reacting in vitro nucleated peripheral blood cells with specific antisera by means of which the known variants are defined. An efficient typing system has been established in many countries for the purposes of organ transplantation and of this already existing system use might be eventually made also for mutation studies.

2) The HL-A genes seem to be expressed without interallelic or intergenic interactions so that the relationship between the genotype and phenotype is desirably simple.

3) The level of heterozygosity at the HL-A gene loci is relatively high which is advantageous for not only gain but also loss mutations to be detectable. In a homozygote, a loss mutation would not be detectable because a simple gene dosage is sufficient for a positive reaction with the specific test reagent to be found. On the other hand a gain mutation might escape detection in a homozygote only on the rather unlikely condition that the gained antigen would be identical with that controlled by the other allele.

4) The major histocompatibility gene complexes in man and mouse

display a great deal of similarity; this provides the advantage that various ancillary experiments may be carried out in mice and help to elucidate questions not directly approachable in man.

Unfortunately, there are also several serious disadvantages of H-systems and in addition, some of the above listed advantages may not hold generally.

First of all, the number of H-loci in a species cannot be estimated with any precision. In mouse, the minimum estimate is 40, but even the figure of over 700 (mutational sites) is compatible with some experimental data (Bailey 1970). Consequently, the mutation rate cannot be expressed on a per locus basis and the observed mutations have to be treated as occurring within a group of loci (similarly as with lethals).

Another and a more serious disadvantage is that for some reason as yet obscure, attempts at inducing H-gene mutations by irradiation failed although the conditions seemed to be most favourable for both induction and detection (Godfrey & Searle 1963, Bailey & Kohn 1965). The latter authors found that the effect – if any – of an acute X-irradiation (522 R) to spermatogonia was to decrease the spontaneous mutation rate in mice (which was 1.35×10^{-2} per zygote). An unexpected finding was a great preponderance of gain-type mutations (i.e. histocompatibility changes which resulted in a new antigen being gained without a former being lost). One possible explanation was that in the tested F_1 hybrids between two inbred strains the chance to *detect* gain mutations was much greater than for loss mutations. This would be so if the about 30 H-loci at which the two parental strains differed represented just a small minority of the existing mutational sites. Another possibility which was considered by the authors was that it was the probability of *inducing* gain type mutations which was much higher. When additional factors were taken into account some kind of correlation was indicated. Under environmental conditions conducive to infection in which the parents of the tested hybrids were conceived and raised, the spontaneous mutation rate seemed to be much higher (0.072) than in the most restrictive environment (0.006). The best interpretation the authors could offer was that the detected histocompatibility changes might have been due rather than to regular mutations to incorporation of viral genomes into the germ line cells of the parents on a principle akin to lysogeny. This could explain the preponderance of gain type variants as well as their reduced frequency among the offsprings of irradiated males (which might be accounted for by a higher radiosensitivity of cells with incorporated viral genomes).

One of the detected spontaneous mutants was submitted to complementation and serological analysis (Bailey et al. 1971). It turned out that although it occurred at the major mouse histocompatibility locus (H-2), it could not be defined serologically, but only by transplantation tests. Thus, the expectation of an easy serological detectability of new H-gene variants, which was listed above among the potential advantages, need not be necessarily fulfilled. Egorov et al. (1972) who administered repeatedly a chemical mutagen (diethylsulphate) succeeded in inducing two H-2 mutations. One of them which was analyzed in great detail turned out to have resulted in both serologically- and lymphocyte-defined antigenic changes of gain and loss types (Egorov 1974).

The obvious difference between radiation and chemical mutagenesis as observed with H-genes might be due to a difference in the kind of mutations induced by the two types of agents. One would have to assume further that the radiation-specific class of H-gene mutations are incompatible with survival and therefore non-detectable. Some indications that there might be something peculiar about certain H-gene variants come from the failures of immunoselection of true H-2 loss variants of cells grown in vitro. Whereas in H-2 heterozygous tumours, variants readily arise which lack H-2 antigens derived from one parent, loss of both parental H-2 antigens has never been detected.

One probable source of problems concerning mutations of major H-systems is the incomplete understanding of their genetic fine structure which is obviously fairly complex. The present models are based almost exclusively on serological analysis of the detected genetic variants and recombinants and on the assumption of one antibody – one antigen ratio and one antigen – one genetic determinant ratio. Since the same reaction patterns may be equally satisfactorily explained on the one antigen – multiple antibodies principle (Hirschfeld 1965), the genetic models are necessarily affected by the arbitrary interpretation in genetic terms of the serological reactions on which they rest. It has been pointed out that the present data concerning the antigenic polymorphism of the HL-A system are equally compatible with a few or with many structural genes (Bodmer 1972) or with polymorphism of regulatory rather than structural genes (Bodmer 1973). In addition, some seemingly new antigens might be of recombinational rather than mutational origin.

There are some recent data which indicate that the expression of cellular antigens tends to be controlled by other, even unlinked genes (Bias et al. 1974, Boubelik et al. 1975); thus another assumption, namely that of a virtually co-dominant inheritance of H-antigens, which was listed above as one of their potential advantages, may have some exceptions not negligible in practice.

These are obvious sources of uncertainty which make the suitability of H-systems for monitoring the mutation rate in the human population greatly questionable. Nevertheless, they should not be eliminated altogether before having been tested in combination with a number of other systems for monitoring the effect of exposure to chemical mutagens in model experiments on laboratory animals, preferentially mice. A single, relatively simple transplantation test for incompatibility within an originally compatible population of inbred mice (or F_1 hybrids) can reveal a spontaneous or induced mutation at one of numerous gene loci spread more or less randomly throughout the whole genome; as an ancillary indicator, this probably deserves consideration in spite of the other obvious disadvantages.

REFERENCES

Bailey, D. W.: Four approaches to estimating number of histocompatibility loci. Transplant. Proc. 2,32 (1970)

Bailey, D. W., Kohn, H. I.: Inherited histocompatibility changes in progeny of irradiated and unirradiated inbred mice. Genet. Res. (Camb.) 6,330 (1965)

Bailey, D. W., Snell, G. D., Cherry, M.: Complementation and serological analysis of an H-2 mutant. Proc.Symp.Immunogenetics of the H-2 system, Liblice-Prague (1970), pp. 155–162, Karger, Basel (1971)

Bias, W. B., Hopkins, K. A., Hutchinson, J. R., Hsu, S. H.: Evidence for an unlinked gene which modifies HL-A antigen expression. Tissue Antigens 4,36 (1974)

Bodmer, W. F.: Evolutionary significance of the HL-A system. Nature 237,139 (1972)

Bodmer, W. F.: A new genetic model for allelism at histocompatibility and other complex loci: polymorphism for control of gene expression. Transplant.Proc. 5,1471 (1973)

Boubelik, M., Lengerová, A., Bailey, D. W., Matoušek, V.: A model for genetic analysis of programmed gene expression as reflected in the development of membrane antigens. Develop.Biol. (1975)

Egorov, I. K., Blandova Z. K.: Histocompatibility mutations in mice: chemical induction and linkage with the H-2 locus. Genet.Res. (Camb.) 19,133 (1972)

Egorov, I. K.: Genetic control of H-2 alloantigens as inferred from analysis of mutations. Immunogenetics 1,97 (1974)

Godfrey, J., Searle, A. G.: A search for histocompatibility differences between irradiated sublines of inbred mice. Genet.Res. (Camb.) 4,21 (1963)

Hirschfeld, J.: Serological codes: interpretations of immunogenetic systems. Science 148,968 (1965)

THE MONITORING OF HUMAN POPULATIONS FOR MUTATIONS AFFECTING PROTEIN STRUCTURE AND/OR FUNCTION: PROBLEMS AND PROSPECTS[1])

JAMES V. NEEL

This presentation will be devoted to a rather general discussion of the strategy of monitoring germinal mutation rates in man, with particular reference to some recent developments which at the very least should extend our knowledge of the spectrum of mutational effects in man, and at best promises to carry the study of mutation in man to a much more profound level than previously. In this latter regard, I think we will agree that viewed in the context of molecular genetics, the study of both spontaneous and induced mutation in such higher organisms as Drosophila, the mouse, and man remains relatively unsatisfactory. For all three of these organisms, estimates of mutation rates have usually been based on gross phenotypic changes, supplemented, in the same or different experiments, by estimates of the frequency of lethal and deleterious effects. While these approaches have yielded much of value, it has been clear for many years not only that they usually do not define the basic event clearly but may leave much undetected.

At the very outset, let me endorse as strongly as possible the continuing development of test systems with experimental organism, as well as human somatic cell systems. These systems should enable us to screen out of the human environment inexcusably potent mutagens, or, other factors being equal in an industrial setting, choose for further research and development the less potent of two mutagens. However, the very success of these experimental test systems in demonstrating the ubiquity of mutagens in the human environment has in the past and will in the future only increase the demand for attempts to attack the overriding question, of what's happening to germinal mutation rates in man.

[1]) Research supported by ERDA Contract (11-1)-1552.

THE THREE PRINCIPAL APPROACHES TO MONITORING HUMAN POPULATIONS

In general, there are two types of situations under which it might be considered desirable to monitor a human population for an increased mutation rate. The first is that in which a population has been subjected to some insult of finite duration, and the second that in which the population is subjected to a continuing and increasing insult, such as an identifiable increase in some pollutant. In the first instance, one must establish a suitable control population but in the second instance, one can under certain circumstances use the initial portion of the study as control upon the latter. In either case, three principal approaches to the problem may be recognized (Neel, 1972, 1974):

1. The "population characteristics" approach
2. The "sentinel phenotypes" approach
3. The "protein variant" or "molecular" approach.

With the latter two of these methodologies, one can pursue the matter of an increased mutation rate either directly or indirectly. The indirect method does not require family studies; one simply looks for an increase in a phenomenon assumed to be mutational in origin. The direct method, on the other hand, demands family studies, which enable one to say which examples of the phenomenon are due to recent mutation, and seeks to document a greater frequency of this event in the children born to exposed as contrasted to unexposed parents. The direct method is obviously preferable when feasible. With the first approach, only the indirect method is possible.
We will consider the first two of these approaches briefly, and devote the bulk of our attention to the third.

A DISCUSSION OF THE "POPULATION CHARACTERISTICS" APPROACH

1. *Protocol and methodology*

This approach can use as indicators of genetic damage changes in such attributes of the population as abortion rate, stillbirth rate, birth weight, life expectancy, sex ratio, frequency of disease (either at birth or subsequently), and growth and development patterns.

It is clear that all of these indicators may be influenced by many extraneous variables, so that the adequacy of the controls is very critical. Equally critical is constancy in diagnostic standards temporally and across groups. My own experience with this type of approach has been in follow-up studies in Hiroshima and Nagasaki. Here we have relied on two types of controls. The first type consists of children born in Hiroshima and Nagasaki to parents who moved into these two cities subsequent to the bombings. Because of small but potentially meaningful differences in mean age and socioeconomic circumstances between exposed and unexposed parents, we have felt it necessary in these studies to introduce a suitable correction for these variables into any contrasts of children born to radiated and nonradiated parents. The second type of control procedure consists in employing a regression type of analysis wherever possible, contrasting the outcome of births to lightly exposed parents to those to more heavily exposed parents. Even after correction for all identified extraneous variables, we would be very sceptical of an effect which depended for its significance on a contrast between the children of radiated and non-radiated parents, but was not borne out by the regression analysis.

2. An example of the results of this approach

The results of the Hiroshima-Nagasaki study have been summarized on several occasions (Neel and Schull, 1956; Neel, 1963). There was no suggestion of an effect of the radiation exposure on stillbirth rate, birth weight, and frequency of congenital defect, and studies of these indicators were abandoned in 1954. Studies do continue on three other indicators, namely, sex ratio, survival, and growth and development. With respect to sex-ratio, the early data (1946–1955) led us to conclude that "the sex of children born to the survivors of the atomic bombings of Hiroshima and Nagasaki reveals significant changes in the sex ratio of these children, changes in the direction to be expected if exposure had resulted in the induction of sex-linked lethal mutations" (Schull and Neel, 1958). However, subsequent data (1956–1962) did not bear these earlier findings out (Schull, Neel and Hashizume, 1966), and we were left uncertain as to whether a small, early effect had disappeared, or whether there never had been an effect. With the recognition of sex chromosome aneuploids in man in 1959, it was clear that if the effect we had observed was real., it might result from an increase in sex-chromosome non-disjunction as well as from an increase in the rate of mutation resulting in sex-linked lethals (Neel, 1963). Cytogenetic studies of the F_1 born to survivors were initiated in 1966 by Dr. Bloom and Dr. Awa. The results to date, while inconclusive, are in a direction consistent with an increase of sex-chromosome non-disjunction in radiated parents (Awa, Neriishi, Honda, Sofuni, and Hamilton, 1973). The data thus far are much too scanty for a meaningful subdivision along the above-mentioned lines of the sex ratio analysis: the expectation, if these are valid and reinforcing findings, would be for the aneuploids to occur in higher numbers among offspring conceived within the first 10 years following the bombing. Should this finding eventually prove valid, it will lend credibility to the sex-ratio finding – which is another way of saying that even apparently simple surveys must usually be reinforced by careful laboratory studies to meet presentday standards.

The data on survival remain no less equivocal, being consistent with a small effect of paternal radiation but none of maternal, thus corresponding to expectation if in the human radiated female, as in the mouse, the increase in mutant offspring following maternal exposure is largely or entirely confined to a relatively brief period following radiation (Neel, Kato and Schull, 1974). Studies on this important point continue. If indeed mortality rates are increased, no physical basis for the finding is yet apparent. Finally, although the analysis has shown no impairment of growth and development by age 9 months, a study now under way, under the direction of Dr. Furusho, involving the cooperation of the school system, will follow the children through an average age of 10 years. In summary, then, I am glad to say there is no completely convincing suggestion of a genetic effect in the children born to the survivors of the bombings. These results should not only serve to dispel the exaggerated predictions current after the war (and still encountered occasionally but also permit us to begin to set upper bounds on the genetic doubling dose in man (cf. Neel, Kato and Schull, 1974).

I have dwelt on the present status of these studies because even now, 30 years after the bombings, the outcome of the studies on this well defined population, while permitting us to exclude certain results, still remains ambiguous in several areas. The experience also emphasizes that while utilizing population characteristics is the most convenient approach – and all the situation in Hiroshima and Nagasaki permitted 20 years ago – it is an approach with many scientific difficulties. There are also ethical difficulties. The investigator must review his data periodically and present possible findings to his colleagues, yet at the same time not alarm the population of reference by a loose discussion of *possibilities*.

A DISCUSSION OF THE "SENTINEL PHENOTYPE" APPROACH

1. *Protocol and methodology*

This approach depends on certain more or less clearly defined, dominantly inherited phenotypes which are known to arise frequently through mutation and can be diagnosed with little equivocation. One simply defines a study population and follows the children born to members of this population with respect to sporadic cases of such phenotypes as multiple neurofibromatosis, aniridia, epiloia, achondroplasia, bilateral retinoblastoma, Marfan's syndrome, acrocephalosyndactyly, Waardenburg's syndrome, etc. Elsewhere I have considered a protocol which employs a battery of some 12 such phenotypes which collectively arise through mutation with an *estimated* frequency of 50 per 100,000 births (Neel, 1971). Since we do not have a theoretical rate, but an estimate, a monitoring program must take into consideration β or type II errors. Table 1 presents my estimate of the sample sizes necessary to detect increases in the mutation rate of 50 percent, given various arbitrarily set levels of type II errors, i. e., acceptance of false hypothesis. We prefer to work with a value of 0.20 for β. Then, with a one-tailed probability test (for increase in phenomenon), there are required two samples of approximately 121,000 births for a demonstration at the 0.05 probability level, and two samples of approximately 196,000 for one at the 0.01 level. At a crude birth rate of 20 per 1000 population, this entails a reference population of either 6,050,000 or 9,800,000 (for 0.05 and 0.01 probalility levels, respectively), if one wishes to put the study on a year-to-year basis. Vogel (1970) has presented quite similar calculations.
It should be emphasized that no matter how carefully one chooses the phenotypes, some cannot be diagnosed with certainty at birth, and others are complex and require expert judgment for diagnosis.

Table 1: The sample sizes necessary to detect an increase in certain sentinel phenotypes[1].

Value of α	Value of β		
	0.10	0.20	0.49
0.05	167,172	120,688	54,085
t-test	2.89[4]	2.46[3]	1.65[2]
0.01	254,101	195,911	108,136
t-test	3.57[5]	3.13[4]	2.33[3]

[1] From an observed 50 per 100,000 births to 75 per 100,000 births, at the indicated probability levels for Type I (α) and Type II (β) errors. The t-values are based on one-tailed probability distributions.

[2] $0.05 > P > 0.01$

[3] $0.01 > P > 0.005$

[4] $0.005 > P > 0.0005$

[5] $0.0005 > P$

Thus what was loosely termed achondroplasia some 30 years ago now consists of some 11 different syndromes (Rimoin, 1975). This fact requires that rigid diagnostic criteria be established at the outset of any study; one cannot rely on standard reporting procedures to locate cases of interest, but must have a team of expert diagnosticians.

An interesting variant of this approach has recently been suggested by Sugahara and Uyama (1974). Knudsen (1971) has argued that the dominantly-inherited type of retinoblastoma requires the concatenation of a least one somatic mutation in retinal tissue plus the inherited gene, and that sporadic cases result from one or more independent mutations at both the locus mentioned above as involved in germ line mutation plus the locus involved in the somatic mutation. Sugahara and Uyama suggest that an increased mutation rate should be reflected in an earlier age of onset of the tumor and a greater number of independent tumor foci in the retina. Although in theory sound, the validity of the approach is highly dependent on a rigid standardization of diagnostic procedures. For this reason, I doubt if the method can be applied retrospectively.

A DISCUSSION OF THE "PROTEIN VARIANT" APPROACH

1. *Protocol and methodology*

This approach gears the monitoring of mutational events to the search for variant proteins with, then, the necessary family studies to determine whether the variant results from mutation in the preceding, or in a more remote, generation. This approach is rendered feasible by two relatively recent developments. The first is the introduction of relatively inexpensive electrophoretic techniques of high resolving power, beginning with the use of various types of paper as a supporting medium in the early 1950's but perhaps best dated from the introduction of the starch gel method by Smithies in 1955. The second development is the very recent introduction of highly automated, computermanaged analytic apparatus which, synchronizing some 16 reaction chambers in a centrifugal head with a recording spectrophotometer, permits following simultaneously 16 different specimens for reactions based on the kinetic or physical properties of the protein in question, the whole apparatus described by the acronym GEMSAEC (Anderson, 1969). Recently a miniaturized version of this apparatus has been developed which can make determinations on 1–10 μl specimens (Burtis, Mailen, Johnson, Scott, Tiffany and Anderson, 1972) and the first steps have been taken to develop for this machine programs describing kinetic enzyme parameters (Tiffany, Chilcote, and Burtis, 1973). While I have emphasized these two developments, I should mention that there are also others still in the development stages with respect to the detection of variant proteins, some of which we have reviewed elsewhere (Neel, Tiffany and Anderson, 1973). Incidentally, inasmuch as a majority of the electrophoretic variants thus far studied for their kinetic properties have shown departures from the normal, the combination of electrophoretic and kinetic studies should detect overlapping samples of variants. There is an additional point to be emphasized. As the experience with hemoglobin S indicates, a given change in electrophoretic mobility may result from some 30 different amino acid substitutions. In the past, these had to be resolved by the laborious procedures of fingerprinting and amino acid sequence analysis. Now, however, it may be possible to analyze the heterogeneity of a given electrophoretic class by these kinetic studies.

It is suggested that a monitoring program can be built around the examination for variants of a series of proteins of the blood serum and the erythrocyte. Since a major cost in any analysis is the procurement and the preliminary processing of the blood specimen, it will be desirable to examine that specimen for as many proteins as possible. The current state of the art would permit the examination of some 25 proteins which in our hands appear satisfactory for monitoring purposes; it is not unrealistic to expect the number to be doubled in the next 10 years.

While these two approaches will detect a wide-spectrum of protein variation, there is of course much they will not detect. In particular, variants characterized by quantitative effects, such as one might anticipate would result from genetic deletions or from mutations affecting operon-type situations, given the normal wide variation in activity-quantity for many of the proteins and enzymes of the blood, probably cannot be detected with any regularity. Especially in studying radiation effects, where Russell (1965) finds that more than half of the induced mutations are recessive lethals, and hence quite likely due to several different types of gene inactivation or actual physical deletions, this is a serious criticism. On the other hand, from the standpoint of medical impact on populations, recessive lethals, if unaccompanied by heterozygous effects, are far less of a matter for concern than mutations compatible with survival but resulting in marked morbidity.

As for the sentinel phenotypes, so for these types of traits I have in the past made rough calculations concerning the necessary sample sizes. Let us assume that the rate at which spontaneous mutation results in detectable changes in a protein is 0.5×10^{-5} per locus per generation. Let us assume we can monitor for 20 different proteins (some associated, like the α and β chains of hemoglobin) and that we wish to be able, at the 0.05 and 0.01 probability limits, to detect a 50 percent increase in the frequency of mutation. We wish to detect an increase from an estimated 20 per 100,000 births to 30 per 100,000 births. If we accept a Type II (β) error of 0.20 this requires at the 0.05 level some 313,000 person-determinations in each sample or, at the 0.01 level, some 508,000 person-determinations. A Type II error of 0.20 is fairly restrictive, but I have made the calculation at this level on the assumption that one wants to be reasonably certain of not missing a real effect. If the contrasts are to be made annually, employing cord blood, the reference population, at a crude birth rate of 20 per 1000, must be approximately 15,666,000 or 25,430,000 persons. The necessary numbers for different values of β are given in Table 2. If one is content to work on a five-year rather than an annual cycle, which to many, including myself, appears reasonable, then the annual number of determinations and the population base are reduced accordingly.

Table 2: The sample sizes necessary to detect an increase in certain biochemical mutants[1].

Value of α	Value of β		
	0.10	0.20	0.51
0.05	434,012	313,329	135,265
t-test	2.95[4]	2.50[3]	1.65[2]
0.01	659,695	508,603	270,445
t-test	3.64[5]	3.19[4]	2.33[3]

[1] From an observed frequency of 20 per 100,000 births to 30 per 100,000 births, at the indicated probability levels for Type I (α) and Type II (β) errors. The t-values are based on one-tailed probability distributions.

[2] $0.05 > P > 0.01$

[3] $0.01 > P > 0.005$

[4] $0.005 > P > 0.0005$

[5] $0.0005 > P$

It will be noted that the population base which seems necessary to support a program designed to detect a 50 percent increase in mutation rate appears larger for this approach than for the "sentinel phenotype" approach. The difference is primarily due to the fact that the sentinel phenotypes chosen earlier have spontaneous rates which most geneticists would consider relatively high-roughly 2×15^{-5}/generation, whereas in the calculations just submitted, the mutation rate was assumed to be 0.5×10^{-5}/gene/generation. Some recent findings, to which I now turn, have made us suspect 0.5×10^{-5} may be a conservative estimate. If so, then the necessary sample base is less, as it also is if the battery of indicator traits can be substantially increased beyond the 20 assumed in the calculation.

2. The Amerindian study

Our principal experience to date with this molecular approach has been in connection with a rather extensive study of the population genetics of several South American Indian tribes in which we have been engaged the past dozen years. Inter alia, the study has involved obtaining blood specimens from all available members of unselected Indian villages. In addition to the usual genetic typings, these specimens have been surveyed for so-called "private" variants of some 15, usually "monomorphic" serum proteins and erythrocyte enzymes. We find that in a total of 58,469 determinations the average frequency of variants at these 20 loci is either 2.0/1000 determinations or 7.8/1000 determinations (Tanis, Neel, Dovey and Morrow, 1973, and unpublished data), the two such differing figures resulting from the fact that in one of the largest and most extensively studied of the Indian tribes there is a "private" polymorphism of serum albumin (Tanis, Ferrell, Neel and Morrow, 1974). The fact that one variant can have such an impact upon the figures illustrates some of the sampling problems associated with this approach. For Caucasian populations, the frequency of variants for these same 15 proteins is 2.5/1000 determinations (summary in Tanis, Neel, Dovey and Morrow, 1973).

One of the purposes of these determinations has been to estimate an average mutation rate for the structural genes responsible for these proteins, an estimate not only of interest in its own right but ultimately to be compared with similar estimates from other human populations. The studies are still continuing, and we regard the current estimates as quite preliminary. We have employed both the direct and indirect approach to the estimate. The direct approach requires that we assemble father-mother-offspring trios from our data, and check the offspring for the occurrence of a trait not present in either parent. When such a trait is found, the possibility of a discrepancy between alleged and actual parentage must be carefully checked. At last summary (Neel, 1974), we had found no mutations in a total of 30,480 contrasts. This series, of course, has to be extended several-fold before it can begin to yield a significant estimate.

The results of the indirect approach have been somewhat more interesting. On the assumption that the variants we detect are selectively neutral and the population is in equilibrium, we can utilize a formulation due to Kimura and Ohta (1969) to calculate the average mutatoin rate. The assumption of neutrality is a conservative assumption – if more of the mutants tend to be deleterious than favorable, which seems likely, then the mutation rate necessary to maintain the observed numbers is higher. However, in these highly subdivided populations with relatively high infant and childhood mortalities, the role of chance loss outweighs that of a selective loss up to rather considerable selective coefficients. The precise formulation is

$$\mu = \frac{I}{2N} \cdot \frac{1}{\bar{t}_0} \tag{1}$$

where

- I = the average number of mutant alleles per locus among the loci sampled,
- N = the number of individuals in one generation in the population in which ›I‹ has been determined, and
- $\bar{t}_0$ = the average mutant survival time in generations for those mutants not going to fixation.

By definition, ›I‹ should not include those variants that will ultimately go to fixation, but this presumably very small fraction of the total cannot be excluded from any actual data set. The final formula has an appealing simplicity: on the assumption of equilibrium, the mutation rate is equal to the mean proportion of different variants per locus (I/2N) times the fraction of these variants lost each generation ($1/\bar{t}_0$).

This is a deceptively simple equation. The estimation of each of these parameters presents very real difficulties. We have derived an estimate of ›$\bar{t}_0$‹ from a Monte Carlo-type simulation of 4 interrelated Indian villages, for which the input and the life tables and breeding structure are based on our observations of the Yanomama Indians (Li and Neel, 1974). The value is surprisingly small, significantly less than what we would estimate from another formula due to Kimura and Ohta (1969), which relates mutant loss to the "variance effective" N_e. We believe this difference derives from the manner in which the life tables and breeding pattern of the Yanomama depart from the structure implicit in Kimura's formulation. We assume, with some error, that the ›N‹ of reference are the adults of breeding age in a given tribe, and the value of ›I‹ is that derived from this same tribe. Our current estimate of μ based on this approach is 2–3 x 10^{-5}/

gene/generation for electrophoretically detectable variants, and 6–9 x 10^{-5} when the electrophoretically undetectable, „silent" variants are taken into consideration (Neel, 1973).

This seems like a relatively high value, the more so since it encompasses only a part of the mutational spectrum (see above), and may well undergo several revisions. If approximately correct – and if similar values obtain for the types of civilized populations that might be monitored for increased mutation rates – then the feasibility of a monitoring system employing protein indicators is improved, since the necessary sample size is reduced.

4. *Some projections for a Pilot Study in the U. S.*

I would like now to discuss our projections for a small pilot study to test the feasibility of monitoring for increases in mutation rates using the techniques I have been discussing. One does not usually present at an international gathering a study he *hopes* to undertake, but this is a workshop, from which I expect many helpful discussions to come.

I shall assume that we shall soon be able to examine with respect to electrophoretic, kinetic, solubility, and denaturation properties some 30 different proteins found in the blood, at a reasonable cost, and that with the combination of these techniques variants occur with a frequency of 5/1000 examinations. These biochemical developments will significantly reduce the size of the necessary reference population. For the present the electrophoresis will employ starch gel as the supporting medium for all systems, but obviously there is room for a great deal of experimentation as to the most efficient electrophoretic procedures, and an even greater amount of work must be directed towards developing the previously mentioned methodology for detecting variants characterized by alterations of kinetic or physical parameters. But the development of the biochemical techniques may be the least troublesome aspect of any monitoring program. Let me mention five practical problems which must be solved:

a. *Source of blood*

If the monitoring program is to be topical, one needs blood from children. But children don't like venapunctures, and their parents are quite properly protective. Placental blood obtained from the umbilical cord at birth seems the obvious solution to this problem, but it is available for only a brief period in the life cycle, and a repeat specimen is impossible to obtain. Thus if one has exhausted the original sample and wishes to verify a variant, one will almost surely need microtechniques suitable to capillary blood samples.

b. Family studies when a variant is encountered.

Each variant will set off a family study. How best to proceed? I suggest it might be most efficient to obtain specimens from all mothers and fathers while the newborn infant is still in the hospital, the specimen from the father when he comes into the hospital for his first visit to see the new baby. I further suggest one does not study the child's blood until specimens from both parents are at hand. Since clearly one will frequently not obtain specimens from both parents, this implies obtaining many specimens which it will not be necessary to examine, but even so, I believe this is a more efficient approach than attempting to obtain the necessary specimens after the child has left the hospital.

c. Confidentiality of the records

Whenever an apparent mutant is found, the necessary studies must be performed concerning discrepancies between legal and biological parentage. This will presumably be done on stored specimens, so that a special contact with the family will not be necessary. But obviously, any file containing information of this type must be kept highly confidential.

d. Invasion of privacy

Now is a time when the freedom of the scientist to intrude himself into the lives of others is being questioned. We note, for instance, the current discussion in the United States concerning the ethics of surveys for chromosomal abnormalities. Add to this the fact that, as noted above, the study will generate some very personal data, and it seems clear there will be questions of invasion of privacy. I propose a standard written explanation to each parent, the studies only to be undertaken with written permission.

e. Choice of population

At the moment, as hinted above, we contemplate monitoring an unselected series of newborn infants. However, it can be argued that *even* a pilot study should concentrate on high risk groups. Given the well-documented tendency of mutagens also to be carcinogens, at the moment in the U.S. a group of children of unusual interest would be those born to persons occupationally exposed to vinyl chloride (Nelson, 1974).

There are other practical problems, which time does not permit us to pursue. Indeed, in view of the totality of the problem to be overcome by a successful monitoring system, and the financial investment involved, it is not surprising that there are some who are sceptical whether this is the way to go. To these sceptics there is only one answer: geneticists, having created so much concern about the genetic risks of pollution, at this point cannot very well shrink from a serious effort at monitoring – if there's a better way than what we're now discussing, let's consider it.

5. *Combining this type of monitoring with chromosome studies*

I would consider monitoring for chromosome aberrations intermediate in philosophy between the "sentinel phenotype" and the "protein variant" approach, but closer to the latter and, in fact, readily combined with the latter. The same blood sample used for biochemical studies can be utilized for chromosome studies. In fact, since as we shall discuss below, there are bound to be many discussions as to the relevance of these protein variants as indicators of morbidity and mortality from increased mutation rates, it would seem desirable to have parallel cytological studies, since there is usually little ambiguity as to the significance of an abnormal karyogram.

6. *The advantages of this approach for interspecies and somatic-germinal rate comparisons*

One of the problems faced by geneticists in extrapolating from the results of work with experimental organisms to man has been the differences in the indicators of mutation in the various species. Much of this difficulty should disappear if the study of mutation can be carried to the protein level. The structural genes coding for homologous proteins in different species are almost certainly homologous. With cross-species comparisons of mutation rates resulting in gross phenotypes, one can never be certain in any of the species what proportion of the mutational spectrum is being detected, or whether the proportions being detected of each kind of change are comparable. However, with this molecular approach, not only can there be a high degree of specificity in the comparison but, judging from the example set by hemoglobin, it should be possible in selected cases to analyze the mutational event in a structural gene in terms of nucleotide substitutions, minute deletions or duplications, chain termination mutations, or unequal crossing over between chromosomal segments in which tandem duplications occur. In this connection, it should be possible to carry fine structure analysis to the level achieved with hemoglobin for at least three other proteins which are included in our current battery, namely, albumin, carbonic anhydrase I, and transferrin.

In theory, one can develop somatic-cell systems utilizing some of the same protein indicators of mutation rates as are used in the studies of germ cell rates. Since, however, it may be anticipated that with single-cell determinations one will usually kill the cells being examined and so can neither get a repeat determination nor a test of transmissibility of the variant, there will undoubtedly be difficulties in monitoring such cells as erythrocytes or leukocytes for evidences of genetic damage. Clearly, once the conversion factors for extrapolating from somatic cell rates of mutation to those for germinal cells have been established, monitoring of somatic cell rates should largely supersede monitoring of germ cell rates, because of the relative inexpensiveness and convenience of the former.

7. Contribution of this approach to basic genetics

It is clear that a proper program of monitoring man for "molecular" mutations will in the pursuit of its objective yield fascinating data for the population geneticist. At the very least, data will become available concerning the number of rare variants and the frequency of each for a variety of genetic loci, these data lending themselves to a variety of genetic calculations. If in addition eventually mutation rates for individual loci become available, then the study of the interplay between mutation and selection has indeed moved to a more basic level.

We are already quite intrigued by the relatively high frequency of albumin variants in the Amerindian. They constitute almost half of the variants encountered to date. Albumin is a large polypeptide, and on this basis alone might be expected to display a disproportionate number of variants, but is this the sole reason? The fact that total absence of serum albumin is compatible with survival suggests an alternative, that selection again variants at this locus is shomewhat milder than for most other serum proteins and erythrocyte enzymes.

THE COST OF MONITORING

So rapidly is the technology evolving, it is very difficult to cost out a monitoring program. Several years ago I suggested that with automation the examination of each of the two samples of 313,000 person-determinations calculated earlier as necessary to demonstrate a 50 % increase in the mutation rate could be achieved by 40 technicians and 5 supervisory scientists. An equal number of support personnel would be necessary. Those expectations may have been optimistic – let's double the number of persons involved, but also decide to monitor on a five-year cycle. We are talking of an annual budget of several millions – less than the amount spent each year by our National Cancer Institute in testing compounds for their carcinogeneity.

THE COST OF NOT MONITORING

But while the cost of monitoring is considerable, the cost of not monitoring is even greater. Major decisions concerning the development of nuclear energy or the use of pesticides, fungicides, herbicides, or food preservatives are now in abeyance in part because of assumed genetic implications. Given the urgency of these decisions, the costs just mentioned are a small price for the initial steps in building up the factual base for intelligent decisions. I believe it very possible that even extensive studies will reveal no detectable increase in mutation rates. Does this mean the money was wasted? Not at all. While some small increase can never be exluded, at least we will have replaced vague surmise and fear with "upper limit" types of estimates. Conversely, a positive finding will set off a search for an etiological agent, although it must be recognized in the case of the chemical mutagens, finding the responsible agent or agents may not be easy (cf. Neel, 1970).

HOW WELL DO ANY OF THESE APPROACHES SERVE AS INDICATORS OF POPULATION DAMAGE?

Our ultimate concern in these monitoring programs is to evaluate the impact of any increased mutation rate on human morbidity and mortality. A number of distinguished committees have labored mightily at this task but many questions still remain. Currently it is difficult to argue from protein variants to effects on morbidity and mortality in man; I believe that at the same time we are improving our knowledge of the mutational event we will be improving our knowledge of the event's consequences. Even today from such studies as those in Japan we can place limits on the phenotypic effects of an increased mutation rate – limits which will almost surely narrow in the future. Further, if, happily, there is no detectable increase in mutation rates, then there is no impact to be interpreted.

OPPORTUNITIES FOR INTERNATIONAL COLLABORATION

In closing, I should like to emphasize the opportunities for intra- and international collaboration which monitoring programs present. The necessary efforts are such that it would be most unrealistic to expect any one or even several centers to carry the burden of the entire study. Moreover, populations of special interest are to be found in a variety of countries, and it would seem appropriate that each country conduct studies on its own nationals. Hopefully, however, these studies could pursue common protocols, so that the final results can be combined for statistical analysis.

REFERENCES

Anderson, N. G.: Computer interfaced fast analyzers. Science 166, 317–324 (1969)

Awa, A. A., Neriishi, S., Honda, T., Sofuni, T., and Hamilton, H. B.: A cytogenetic survey of the offspring of A-bomb survivors in Hiroshima and Nagasaki, Japan. In: Proceedings, Fourth International Congress on Birth Defects, A. G. Motulsky and F. J. G. Ebling, (Eds.), p. 92. (Excerpta Medica International Congress Series 297.) Amsterdam: Excerpta Medica Press (1973)

Burtis, C. A., Mailen, J. C., Johnson, W. F., Scott, C. D., Tiffany, T. O., and Anderson, N. G.: Development of a miniature fast analyzer. Clin. Chem. 18, 753–761 (1972)

Neel, J. V.: Changing Perspectives on the Genetic Effects of Radiation. Springfield, Ill.: Charles C. Thomas, pp. VIII & 97 (1963)

Neel, J. V.: Evaluation of the effects of chemical mutagens on man: The long road ahead. Proc. Nat. Acad. Sci. (U. S.) 67, 908–915 (1970)

Neel, J. V.: The detection of increased mutation rates in human populations. Perspectives Biol. Med. 14, 522–537 (1971)

Neel, J. V.: "Private" genetic variants and the frequency of mutation among American Indians. Proc. Nat. Acad. Sci. (U. S.) 70, 3311–3315 (1973)

Neel, J. V.: Developments in monitoring human populations for mutation rates. Mutation Res. 26, 319–328 (1974)

Neel, J. V., Kato, H., and Schull, W. J.: Mortality in the children of atomic bomb survivors and controls. Genetics 76, 311–326 (1974)

Neel, J. V., and Schull, W. J.: The Effect of Exposure to the Atomic Bombs on Pregnancy Termination in Hiroshima and Nagasaki. Washington: National Academy of Sciences-National Research Publication 461, pp. XVI and 241 (1956)

Neel, J. V., Tiffany, T. O., and Anderson, N. G.: Approaches to monitoring human populations for mutation rates and genetic disease. In: Chemical Mutagens, Volume 3: Principles and Methods for Their Detection, A. Hollaender, (Ed.), pp, 105–150. New York: Plenum Publishing Corporation (1973)

Kimura, M., and Ohta, T.: The average number of generations until extinction of an individual mutant gene in a finite population. Genetics 63, 701–709 (1969)

Knudson, A. G.: Mutation and cancer: Statistical study of retinoblastoma. Proc. Nat. Acad. Sci. (U. S.) 68, 820–823 (1971)

Li, F.H.F., and Neel, J. V.: A simulation of the fate of a mutant gene of neutral selective value in a primitive population. In: Computer Simulation in Human Population Studies, B. Dyke and J. MacCluer, (Eds.), pp. 221–238. New York, Academic Press (1974)

Rimoin, D. L.: The chondrodystrophics. Adv. Hum. Genet. 5, 1–118 (1975)

Russell, W. L.: Studies in mammalian radiation genetics. Nucleonics 23, 53–62 (1965)

Schull, W. J., and Neel, J. V.: Radiation and the sex ratio in man. Science 128, 343–348 (1958)

Schull, W. J., Neel, J. V., and Hashizume, A.: Some further observations on the sex ratio among infants born to survivors of the atomic bombings of Hiroshima and Nagasaki. Amer. J. Hum. Genet. 18, 328–338 (1968)

Sugahara, T., and Uyama, M.: A possible population monitoring system on environmental mutagens: Statistical studies on retinoblastoma in Japan.

Presentation at Symposium on Mutagenesis and Carcinogenesis sponsored by U. S.–Japan Medical Science Cooperative Program, Tokyo, (1974)

Tanis, R., Ferrell, R. E., Neel, J. V., and Morrow, M.: Albumin Yanomama-2, a 'private' polymorphism of serum albumin. Ann. Hum. Genet., Lond 38, 179–190 (1974)

Tanis, R. J., Neel, J. V., Dovey, H., and Morrow, M.: The genetic structure of a tribal population, the Yanomama Indians. IX. Gene frequencies for 18 serum protein and erythrocyte enzyme systems in the Yanomama and five neighboring tribes: nine new variants. Amer. J. Hum. Genet. 25, 655–676 (1973)

Tiffany, T. O., Chilcote, D. D., and Burtis, C. A.: Evaluation of enzyme kinetic parameters by use of a small computer interfaced "fast analyzer" – an addition to automated clinical enzymology. Clin. Chem. 19, 908–918 (1973)

Vogel, F.: Monitoring of human populations. In: Chemical Mutagenesis in Mammals and Man, F. Vogel and G. Röhrborn, (Eds.), pp. 445–452. Heidelberg, Springer-Verlag (1970)

MICROELECTROPHORESIS FOR RAPID FRACTIONATION OF RNA, PROTEINS, ENZYMES, AND ISOENZYMES

V. NEUHOFF

The necessity of using microchemical methods in brain research is obvious for the analysis of well-defined brain regions or even isolated neurons. On the other hand, micromethods are usually much less time-consuming than the commonly used macromethods so that it is often advantageous to use microtechniques even if the material to be analysed is not limited in quantity. Because the resolution power and the reproducibility in microfractionations is at least as good as in the normal scale the micromethods may very effectively be used in human population monitoring for detection of increased mutation rates. Since in this connection the analysis of RNA, proteins, enzymes, and isoenzymes may be of special interest this lecture will concentrate on a brief description of corresponding micromethods giving some examples for their application.

In general, the correct performance of micromethods is no more arduous than the equivalent macroscale method. Any experimentalist with some experience will be able to learn quickly the handling of these methods and the time necessary to become an expert will be the same as for any method. However, the biggest barrier to moving from the normal to the microscale is often only the experimentalist's scepticism about any method which has been reduced to a microscale.

Electrophoresis on polyacrylamide gels with diameters of 5 or 7 mm is in general used as a laboratory technique for many different fractionation problems (Revue see Maurer, 1971). The first application on a microscale of polyacrylamide gel electrophoresis was carried out in 1964 when Pun and Lombrozo fractionated brain proteins. Since that time the technique has developed very well and is adapted also to many different fractionation problems (Revue see Neuhoff, 1973). Calibrated microcaps with volumes from 1 to 10 μl are routinely used for microdisc electrophoresis or microgradient electrophoresis. Accordingly the diameter of microgels is small (0.2–0.6 mm) allowing one to perform the staining procedure in 5 min and the decolourizing process in about 30 min. The lower limit of detection for a single protein band in a 5 μl gel of 0.45 mm diameter is 10^{-9} g of albumin when visualized with amido black 10B. 0.1–0.5 μg of a protein mixture can be fractionated by electrophoresis in capillaries, meaning that 5000–10 000 fractionations can be performed with 1 ml solution containing 1 mg protein. The duration of electrophoresis depends on the type of protein to be fractionated, but is generally between 20 and 60 min.

Microdisc electrophoresis is normally performed on homogeneous polyacrylamide gels of 10–20 % acrylamide concentration with 2 % cross-linking. The sample gel has to be overlayered by a 5 % collecting gel. (For technical details of gel preparation stock solutions, gel handling etc. see Neuhoff, 1973). The optimal concentration of a solution for fractionation is 1–3 mg protein/ml. More concentrated solutions must be diluted, since the capacity of the gel for separation is easily exhausted by overloading. The progress of electrophoresis can be followed either on the voltage generator (Neuhoff et al., 1967) for each of 10 individual capillaries or by observing the migration of bromophenol blue or bromophenol red which is added to the sample before fractionation. Immediately after electrophoresis, routinely performed at 60–80 Volt, the gels are expelled from the capillaries by water pressure derived from a syringe. This creates no problems since the gel mixture contains Triton X-100. For routine evaluation, pherograms of the gels are recorded by means of a microdensitometer in a special glass chamber (Neuhoff, 1968). Recently, Zimmer and Neuhoff (1975) have described equipment allowing evaluation of microgels at any suitable wave length using a spectrophotometer. Isolation of individual protein fractions after an initial fractionation in a microgel for a second fractionation or for a microimmunoassay is described by Neuhoff and Schill (1968). After microdialysis (Neuhoff and Kiel, 1969) isolated protein fractions can also be used for determining the amino acid composition or the C- and N-terminal amino acids (Neuhoff et al., 1970).

Application of microdisc electrophoresis to enzyme analysis

Microanalysis of DNA-dependent DNA and RNA polymerase. The enzymatically active components of a preparation of DNA-dependent DNA or RNA polymerase can be characterized using two basically different methods. These are the *binding test,* which gives an indirect characterization and the *polymerisation test* which gives direct cha-

racterization (Neuhoff and Lezius, 1967, 1968). For the binding test two parallel runs are performed. One gel capillary is loaded only with the enzyme preparation under investigation and a second identical gel capillary is loaded first with a layer of DNA or poly d(A-T) solution as the template and afterwards with the same quantity of enzyme solution as used in the first capillary. During electrophoresis the polymerase particles have to pass through the layer of template solution thereby forming a complex with the primer which scarcely migrates into the separating gel. On staining with amido black after electrophoresis, the active protein components of the polymerase are not detected in the gel. By comparing this gel with that on which the enzyme preparation was directly fractionated, a clear differentiation between the enzymatically active and inactive protein components of the fractionated solutions can be made. Using the same method, a series of binding tests can be made for testing the influence of individual components, e.g. the effect of different substrates or ions on the formation of the enzymetemplate complex (Neuhoff and Lezius, 1968).
For the *polymerisation test* a suitable amount of the primer, DNA or poly d(A-T) is added to the gel mixture and the capillaries are filled with this mixture as usual. In this way the same concentration of primer is present throughout the gel. The 5 % collecting gel is added and the preparation of polymerase is fractionated in the 'primer-gel' as before. After electrophoresis the gels are placed in a mixture of suitable substrates (depending on the primer in the gel) and incubated for defined time intervals and thereafter the synthesized product is visualized by staining with pyronine or toluidine blue. The evaluation is performed by planimetry of microdensitometer tracings. Neuhoff et al. (1968, 1969a,b, 1970) have used both methods for analysis and characterization of DNA-dependent RNA-polymerase from E.coli.

Quantitative assay for dehydrogenases

Microdisc electrophoresis of dehydrogenases (Cremer et al., 1972) is usually performed in 5 μl capillaries on normal gel systems. (For details see Neuhoff, 1973.) One of the advantages of this micromethod is its high sensitivity for the determination of different dehydrogenases; it is at least 1000 times more sensitive than a common photometric test. The minimum amount of pure glucose-6-phosphate dehydrogenase (Glc-6-P DH) from yeast which can be detected after amido black staining after fractionation on 20 % polyacrylamide gels in 5 μl capillaries is approximately 1 ng, as compared to the ease of activity measurements, using amounts of less than 1 pg of yeast Glc-6-P DH, with the tetrazolium assay (Brewer and Sing, 1970; Wilkinson, 1970). Because of the small diameter of the microgels, the time of diffusion of the substrates into the gel is so low that a linear increase in optical density can be observed at the site of enzymic activity in the gel, after two or three minutes of incubation in the assay mixture. This linear increase can be followed for a period of between 15 and 80 min, depending on the enzyme concentration, showing that only negligible amounts of enzyme are lost from the gel during incubation. It is, therefore, possible to compare a microgel to a "Micro-cuvette" with a volume from 0.003 to 0.015 μl, since a single protein band in a 5 μl gel extends approximately 20 to 100 μm. The blue formazan, which is the final product of the coupled reactions, remains as a precipitate at the site of enzymic activity in the gel and can be recorded during incubation densitometrically. The method can be standardized in international units by using enzyme preparations of known activity. Cremer et al. (1972) have shown that the method is equally suitable for the separation of enzyme variants by assaying their enzymic activity in an 'one-step' procedure and also that Michaelis-Menten kinetic can be performed using microgels (Endou and Neuhoff, 1975).

When enzymes are used as markers for genetic analysis it is often necessary to characterize an enzyme by determination of several parameters. Therefore, the calculation of binding constants for the enzymes, even in polyacrylamide microgels, may be advantageous. For further characterization the effect of activators or inhibitors can also be investigated. The well known cycling method described by Lowry et al. (1961), and Lowry and Passonneau (1972) is more sensitive than the method described here. However, for genetic problems enzyme variants which are used as genetic markers, have to be separated prior to identification. Such work, therefore, requires methods which are not only sensitive but which can also separate variants of enzymes. The micro-assay of dehydrogenases in polyacrylamide microgels meets these two requirements.

Microisoelectric focussing

Haglund (1971) described in a comprehensive review the historical development, the theoretical foundations and the applications at the macroscale level of this very important and powerful method of protein fractionation. Applications to the microscale level are reported by Riley and Coleman (1968), Catsimpoolas (1968), Quentin and Neuhoff (1972), Gainer (1973) and Grossbach (1974). Quentin and Neuhoff (1972) have combined isoelectric focussing of isoenzymes in 5 μl capillaries with enzyme activity measurements of the separated isoenzyme using the tetrazolium assay. For example, only μg amounts of tissue are necessary for determining the activity of LDH isoenzymes quantitatively.

Microelectrophoresis on Gradient gels

Gradient gel electrophoresis has proved to be useful for various separations on the macroscale (Revue see Maurer, 1971). The simplest method for production of polyacrylamide gradients in microcapillaries with an inner diameter lower than 1 mm is given by Rüchel et al. (1973) using only capillary attraction. The specially cleaned capillaries are filled by dipping them into appropriate solutions. In this way, the gel components are continuously mixed, to give a linear gradient of concentration in the polymerized gel between 1.2 % acrylamide at the top of the gel and approximately 50 % at the bottom. The length and steepness of the gradient can be varied, as can the range of concentration, so that the gradient can be adapted to the problem of fractionation.

The fractionation on polyacrylamide gradient gel can replace microdisc electrophoresis for many different separations since it gives a sharper separation of the proteins and the manipulations required are simpler. For example, the cumbersome preparation of a 5 % collecting gel is not necessary. By varying the method of producing the gradient, the application of the sample can also be performed by capillary attraction, thus avoiding the use of micropipettes. This procedure appears to be very suitable for routine laboratory analyses, something which cannot be said, without further qualification, for microdisc electrophoresis. The limits of detectability for individual protein bands in a gradient gel, the sample volumes to be fractionated and the quantities of protein contained in them are identical with those for microdisc electrophoresis. Polyacrylamide gradient gels have the further advantage that, owing to the high acrylamide concentration at the lower end, they can be pushed from the capillaries with a well-fitting steel wire without damaging the gel section where separation has taken place. The presence of Triton X-100 can be avoided in the gel mixture thus allowing SDS in microscale gel electrophoresis (Rüchel et al., 1974).

As an example of the high resolution power of microgradient gels Fig. 1 shows the fractionation of a mixture of proteins with molecular weights ranging from 10^4 to 10^7. Electrophoresis on microgradient gels

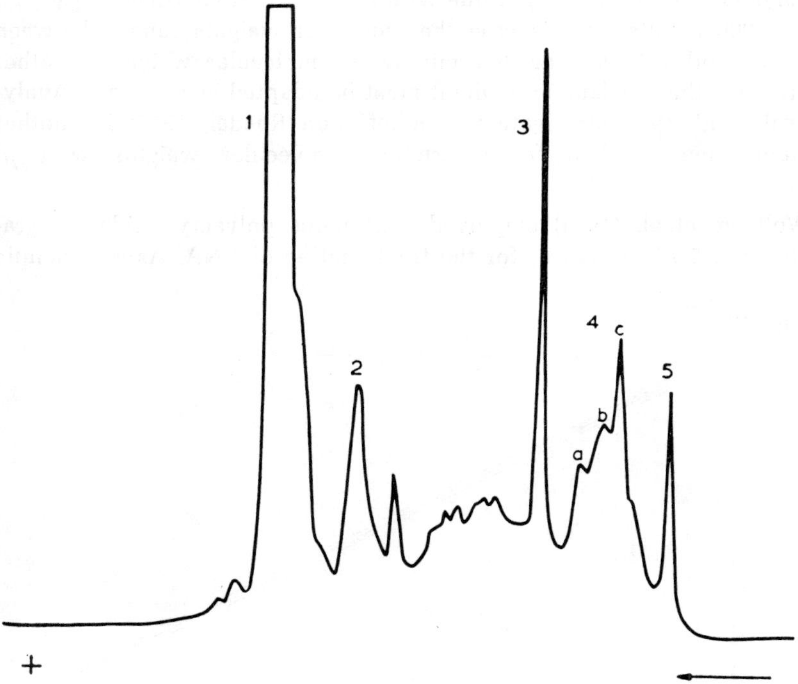

Fig. 1: Fractionation (30 min, 60 Volt) of a mixture of human serum, ribosomes from rabbit reticulocytes and Friend-virus particles in a 5 µl gradient-gel.

Peak 1: Human albumin (MW 69 000). The shoulder derives from calf serum of the virus preparation. Peak 2: Transferrin (MW 88 000), Peak 3: $_2$-macroglobulin from the human serum (MW 900 000), Peak 4a: 40 S ribosomal subunit (MW 1.3×10^6), Peak 4b: 60 S ribosomal subunit (MW 2.8×10^6), Peak 4c: 80 S subunit (MW 4.2×10^6), Peak 5: virus particle (MW approx. 1×10^7).

(From Rüchel, Mesecke, Wolfrum, Neuhoff 1973)

can also be used to determine molecular weights of proteins as shown in Fig. 2. A preparation of 100 % pure crystalline human albumin, containing several polymeric forms of albumin, was used for this fractionation on a 5 μl gradient gel. After staining with amido black the relative mobilities were determined from the respective microdensitometer curves. If the relative mobility is plotted against the logarithm of the molecular weights of albumin and the four visible polymeric forms, a straight line with a correlation coefficient $r_{lgMW\ mm} = 1.000$ results. In this case the molecular weights ranged between 67.000 and 335.000. For determining the molecular weights of other proteins, the acrylamide gradient must be adapted accordingly. Analytical capillary centrifugation (Neuhoff and Roedel, 1973) is another independent method for determining molecular weights with μl samples.

Wolfrum et. al. (1974) employed continuous polyacrylamide gel gradients in 5 μl capillaries for the fractionation of RNA. As an example

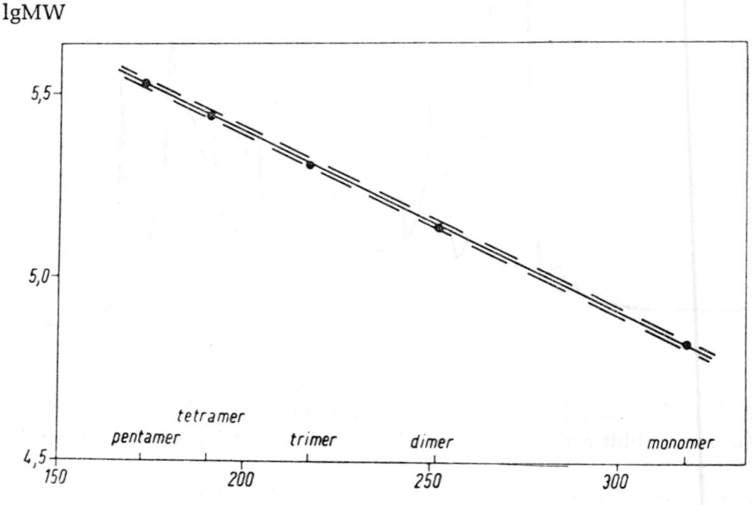

Fig. 2: Plot of the relative migration distance against the logarithms of the molecular weights of albumin and its polymeric forms after fractionation in a 5 µl polyacrylamide gradient gel.
(From Rüchel, Mesecke, Wolfrum, Neuhoff 1973)

fig. 3 shows a densitogram after fractionation and toluidin blue staining of a mixture of different RNA species. As a further example of the very high resolution power of microgradient gels fig. 4 shows densitograms after fractionation and toluidin blue staining of different mixtures of $tRNA^{Phe}$. Using polyacrylamide gradient microelectrophoresis it is possible to separate tRNAs in the pmole range which differ only in one nucleotide in length and allow their rapid and reproducible characterization. Separation of aminoacyl-tRNA from the uncharged molecule is also possible by this method, which allows its identification without using radioactive labels (Sprinzl et al., 1975).

Autoradiography of microgels

The autoradiography of microgels prepared in microcapillaries is of particular interest for recording, e.g. incorporation in or binding of radioactive substances to proteins or RNA. Placing the round, moist microgels on a sensitive X-ray film is unsatisfactory both because the small area for contact and because the gels dry out and shrink unevenly during the time of exposure. Both drawbacks are eliminated by freezedrying the microgels before autoradiography (Neuhoff et al., 1973). The gels can be initially stained and evaluated microdensitometrically.

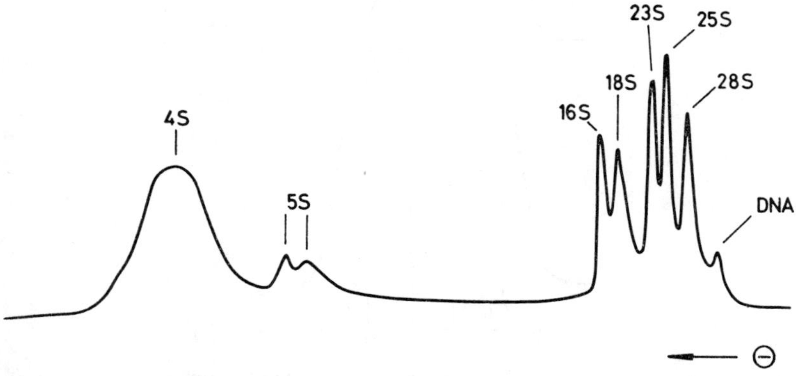

Fig. 3: Densitogram after fractionation of a mixture of RNA from rat brain (28 S, 18 S, 5 S, 4 S), pea seedling root tips (25 S, 18 S, 5 S, 4 S), E.coli (23 S, 16 S, 5 S, 4 S) and tRNA from yeast in a 5 µl gradient gel with a slope from 1–40 % acrylamide concentration.
(From Wolfrum, Rüchel, Mesecke, Neuhoff 1974)

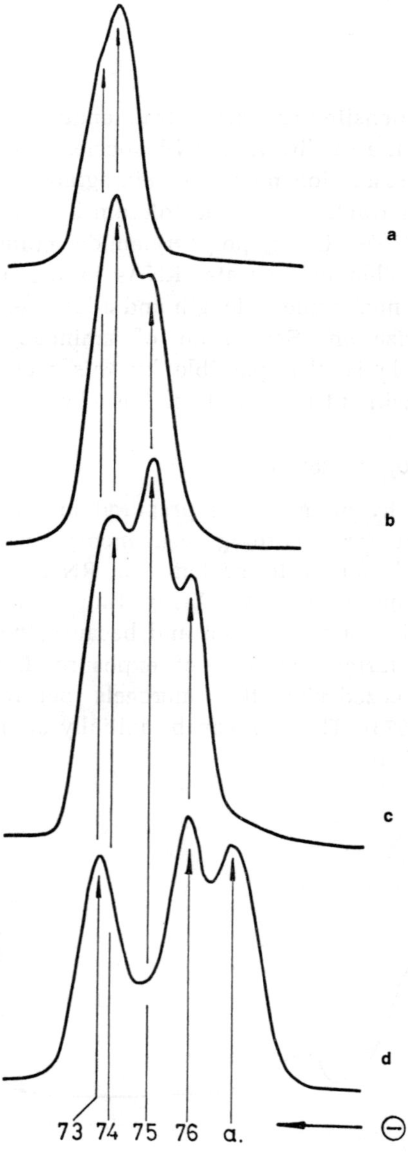

Fig. 4: Separation of different mixtures of $tRNA^{Phe}$. The number of the peaks corresponds with the number of the 3'-end nucleotide of the tRNA. a. indicates the position of the aminoacylated tRNA.

a) $tRNA^{Phe}$-A_{73} + $tRNA^{Phe}$-C_{74}

b) $tRNA^{Phe}$-C_{74} + $tRNA^{Phe}$-C_{75}

c) $tRNA^{Phe}$-C_{74} + $tRNA^{Phe}$-C_{75} + $tRNA^{Phe}$-A_{76}

d) $tRNA^{Phe}$-A_{73} + $tRNA^{Phe}$-A_{76} + Phe-$tRNA^{Phe}$C-C-3'NH_2A.

(From Sprinzl, Wolfrum, Neuhoff 1975)

The examples described serve to show that practically all fractions which are performed on polyacrylamide gels on the macroscale can also be carried out with microelectrophoresis. For some applications, e. g. for investigations of enzyme kinetics, the micromethod has a distinct advantage, and indeed may be the only possible method of analysis, owing to the short distance for diffusion in the microgels. An experienced experimentalist conversant with the techniques described in full detail by Neuhoff (1973) should find it easy to adapt microelectrophoresis on polyacrylamide gels to any specific problem of separation.

REFERENCES

Brewer, G.J. and Sing, C.F.: An introduction to Isoenzyme Techniques, Academic Press, New York, London (1970)

Catsimpoolas, N.: Micro isoelectric focussing in polyacrylamide gel columns. Analyt.Biochem. 26, 480–482 (1968)

Cremer, Th., Dames, W. and Neuhoff, V.: Micro disc electrophoresis and quantitative assay of glucose-6-phosphate dehydrogenase at the cellular level. Hoppe-Seyler's Z. Physiol.Chem. 353, 1317–1329 (1972)

Endou, H. and Neuhoff, V.: Kinetic studies of microsomal glucose dehydrogenase in rat liver. Hoppe-Seyler's Z. Physiol. Chem., 356, 1381–1396 (1975)

Grossbach, U.: Micro disc electrophoresis in capillary columns, in: Electrophoresis and Isoelectric Focussing in Polyacrylamide Gel (Ed. R.C. Allen and H.R. Maurer) Walter de Gruyter, Berlin, New York, pp. 207–213 (1974)

Haglund, H.: Isoelectric focussing in pH gradients. A technique for fractionation and characterization of ampholytes, in: Methods of Biochemical Analysis (Ed. D. Glick), Vol. 19, Wiley Interscience, New York, London, Sydney, Toronto, pp. 1–104 (1971)

Lowry, O.H. and Passonneau, J.V.: A Flexible System of Enzymatic Analysis, Academic Press, New York (1972)

Maurer, H.R.: Disc electrophoresis and related techniques of polyacrylamide gel electrophoresis, Walter de Gruyter, Berlin, New York (1971)

Neuhoff, V.: Micro-Disc-Electrophorese von Hirnproteinen. Arzneimittel-Forsch. 18, 35–39 (1968)

Neuhoff, V.: Micromethods in Molecular Biology, in: Molecular Biology, Biochemistry and Biophysics, Vol. 14 (Eds. A. Kleinzeller, G.F. Springer und H.G. Wittmann), Springer Verlag, Berlin, Heidelberg, New York (1973)

Neuhoff, V. and Kiehl, F.: Dialysiergeräte für Volumen zwischen 10 und 500 µl. Arzneimittel-Forsch. (Drug.Res.) 19, 1898–1899 (1969)

Neuhoff, V. and Lezius, A.: Nachweis der Struktur von DNA-Polymerasen, der enzymatisch aktiven Proteinkomponente und ihrer Enzym-Substrat-Komplexe mit der Micro-Disc-Electrophorese. Hoppe-Seyler's Z.Physiol. Chem. 348, 1239 (1967)

Neuhoff, V., Mühlberg, B. and Meier, J.: Strom- und spannungskonstantes Netzgerät für die Micro-Disc-Elektrophorese. Arzneimittel-Forsch. 17, 649–651 (1967)

Neuhoff, V. and Rödel, E.: Analytische Kapillarzentrifugation. Hoppe-Seyler's Z. Physiol.Chem. 354, 1541–1549 (1973)

Neuhoff, V. and Schill, W.-B.: Kombinierte Mikro-Disk-Elektrophorese und Mikro-Immunpräzipitation von Proteinen. Hoppe-Seyler's Z. Physiol. Chem. 349, 795–800 (1968)

Neuhoff, V., Schill, W.-B., Sternbach, H.: Mikro-Disk-electrophoretische Analyse reiner DNA-abhängiger RNA-Polymerase aus *Escherichia coli.* I. Struktur und Matrizenabhängige Funktion. Hoppe-Seyler's Z. Physiol. Chem. 349, 1126–1136 (1968)

Neuhoff, V., Schill, W.-B. and Sternbach, H.: Mikro-Disk-elektrophoretische Analyse reiner DNA-abhängiger RNA-polymerase aus *Escherichia coli.* III. Differenzierung zwischen Syntheseort und Bindungsort für die Matrize. Hoppe-Seyler's Z. Physiol.Chem. 350, 335–340 (1969a)

Neuhoff, V., Schill, W.-B. and Sternbach, H.: Mikro-Disk-elektrophoretische Aanlyse reiner DNA-abhängiger RNA-Polymerase aus *Escherichia coli.* IV. Isolierung und Charakterisierung elektrophoretisch getrennter Enzymfraktionen. Hoppe-Seyler's Z. Physiol. Chem. 350, 767–774 (1969b)

Neuhoff, V., Schill, W.-B. and Sternbach, H.: Micro-analysis of pure deoxyribonucleic-acid-dependent ribonucleic acid polymerase from *Escherichia coli.* Action of heparin and rifampicin on structure and function. Biochem.J. 117, 623–631 (1970)

Neuhoff, V., Weise, M. and Sternbach, H.: Micro-analysis of pure deoxyribonucleic acid-dependent ribonucleic acid polymerase from *Escherichia coli.* VI. Determination of the amino acid composition. Hoppe-Seyler's Z.Physiol.Chem. 351, 1395–1401 (1970)

Quentin, C.-D. and Neuhoff, V.: Micro-isoelectric focussing for the detection of LDH isoenzymes in different brain regions of rabbit. Int.J.Neurosci. 4, 17–24 (1972)

Riley, R.F. and Coleman, M.K.: Isoelectric fractionation of proteins on a microscale in polyacrylamide and agarose matrices. J.Lab.clin.Med. 72, 714–720 (1968)

Rüchel, R., Mesecke, S., Wolfrum, D.-I. and Neuhoff, V.: Mikroelektrophorese an kontinuierlichen Polyacrylamid-Gradientengelen, I. Herstellung und Eigenschaften von Gelgradienten in Kapillaren; ihre Anwen-

dung zur Proteinfraktionierung und Molekulargewichtsbestimmung. Hoppe-Seyler's Z.Physiol.Chem. 354, 1351–1368 (1973)
Rüchel, R., Mesecke, S., Wolfrum, D.-I., and Neuhoff, V.: Micro-electrophoresis in continuous-polyacrylamide-gradient gels. II. Fractionation and dissociation of sodium dedecylsulphate protein complexes. Hoppe-Seyler's Z. Physiol.Chem. 355, 997–1020 (1974)
Sprinzl, M., Wolfrum, D.-I. and Neuhoff, V.: Separation of Aminoacyl-$tRNA^{Phe}$ and $tRNAs^{Phe}$ with partially hydrolysed 3'-end by polyacrylamide gradient Micro-electrophoresis. FEBS LETTERS 50, 54–56 (1975)
Wilkinson, J.H.: Isoenzymes, 2nd.edn. Chapman and Hill, London (1970)
Wolfrum, D.-I., Rüchel, R., Mesecke, S. and Neuhoff, V.: Mikroelektrophorese in kontinuierlichen Polyacrylamid-Gradientengelen. III. Extraktion und Fraktionierung von Ribonucleinsäuren im Mikromaßstab. Hoppe-Seyler's Z. Physiol. Chem. 355, 1415–1435 (1974)
Zimmer, H.-G. and Neuhoff, V.: Photometrie von Mikrogelen. G-I-T Fachzeitschrift für das Laboratorium 19, 481–484 (1975)

PRIORITIES IN ASSESSING THE IMPACT ON HUMAN POPULATIONS OF AN INCREASED MUTATION RATE

HOWARD B. NEWCOMBE

The past few years have seen an upswing in interest, on the part of many geneticists, in the possible harmful effects on human health and well-being of an increase in mutation rate due to the widerspread use of chemical compounds which may have mutagenic properties. Geneticists are understandably anxious to test in the laboratory various food additives, drugs, insecticides, and pollutants, to determine which of them might be acting to raise the mutation rate in man. If it were just a matter of deciding which compounds are bad, and of thereafter discontinuing their use, this kind of effort on the part of geneticists should be sufficient to settle the matter.

But if a drug or an insecticide, for example, has positive value for society, some will argue that its use should be continued unless its mutagenic effects can be shown to represent a substantial threat to human health. Thus, much depends on the ability of geneticists to say something useful about the magnitude of the harm which mutations can cause.

Let us suppose, to take an extreme example, that laboratory tests had indicated that current levels of a particular mutagenic chemical were sufficient to double the mutation rate in man. Geneticists would almost certainly be pressed to say whether the effects on human health were likely to be important, or trivial. The answer to this question will not be found in the results of studies on mutation induction. Knowing the numbers of mutations produced does not tell us how much additional disease will occur. And if geneticists are seriously worried by the social problems about which they voice concern, they will, in the near future, shift some major part of their research effort into this particular gap in genetic knowledge. Otherwise, ignorance on the point will make the results of their mutation studies largely uninterpretable.

A number of relevant areas of uncertainty that have so far failed to attract sufficient attention deserve special mention:

a) One of these has to do with the magnitude of the social burden from hereditary disease. Geneticists regard the hereditary component in human ill health as important, but surprisingly little effort has been devoted to assessing the total impact of genetic disease. There are a few estimates of the total frequencies of the hereditary and partially hereditary diseases of man (Stevenson 1959, Trimble and Doughty 1974) but little information on the social cost of these diseases in terms, for example, of the burden they place on the health services or the economy of a country.

b) What is more important is that we have little evidence concerning the role of the natural mutation rate in determining the prevalence of the diseases. Geneticists are reasonably certain that the frequencies of the simple dominant conditions, such as retinoblastoma and achondroplastic dwarfism, are maintained by new mutations in each generation. The serious dominant diseases were at one time believed to affect one child out of every 100 born alive; so that a doubling of the mutation rate used to be regarded as probably doubling that 1 per cent. But a recent estimate of the frequency of simple dominant disease, based on new data, is ten-fold lower, i.e. one case per 1000 born alive, instead of one per 100 (Trimble and Doughty 1974). This observation reduces ten-fold the predicted amount of dominant disease that would result from a doubling of the mutation rate, but it tells us nothing about the effect on the vastly more numerous and important irregularly inherited diseases, many of which are multifactorial in origin.

c) The less regularly inherited conditions such as diabetes, epilepsy, cleft palate, and pyloric stenosis, are perhaps 50 times as common as the simple dominant diseases, and yet we know virtually nothing about the role that mutation may, or may not, play in determining their prevalence. What is even more serious in the present context is that few geneticists are interested in studying the problem. It has sometimes been suggested that perhaps a third of the irregularly inherited diseases might be mutation-maintained. But this is pure guess-work. No one has demonstrated empirically that any known irregularly inherited disease of mice, such as cleft palate for example, undergoes any increase at all following generations of repeated irradiation. There is, in fact, little interest in carrying out such studies because the experiments that have already been done have yielded largely negative results, so that the approach is regarded as scientifically dull and professionally unrewarding. And yet, how else can one hope to equate changes in mutation frequency with changes in the incidence of a broad category of hereditary disease that seriously affects at sometime in their lives at least 5 individuals out of every 100 born alive?

The purpose of this discussion is to remind those who are busy in the laboratory screening various environmental contaminants for mutagenic activity, that the results from their labours may remain largely without meaning if they cannot relate, in some quantitative fashion, numbers of mutations with numbers of sick people. If geneticists are, in fact, serious about the possible social importance of environmental mutagens, they will soon begin strengthening this weakest link in their chain of reasoning.

The relevant human studies are not without theoretical interest. For the great bulk of the hereditary and partially hereditary diseases of man we have almost no idea whether mutation, or selection, determines the prevalence of the causal genes. Current theory is of little help because there are competing theories which favour opposite conclusions. This is why it is so difficult to say whether even a sustained doubling of the mutation rate would have an important, or just a trivial, effect on human health.

In planning our own research program at Chalk River it was decided some time ago that the human data required for the relevant studies had to be more extensive than those normally obtained by means of ad hoc investigations of conventional design and scope. It seemed that if society were truly faced with genetic problems as important as some had claimed, and in fact still claim, the manner and scale of the extraction of human data ought properly to reflect the magnitude of the concern that was being expressed. To answer some of the important questions might well require systematic use of information on disease and family relationships for whole populations of substantial size. Our own efforts in this direction have made use of a number of the large files of health related records that are generated routinely in the Canadian province of British Columbia, which has a present population of two and a quarter million people.

Individuals do leave behind them, as they proceed through life, a more extensive trail of paper documentation than they care to think about. Family relationships are recorded for legal purposes whenever people are born, get married, produce children, or die. Information about their health is likewise recorded at birth, when they are hospitalized or visit a physician's office, when they die, and also in various specialized registers of cancer and of other serious conditions such as congenital malformations and various handicapping diseases. To an increasing extent this information is finding its way into computers which are capable of handling very large files.

For the purpose of studying the total burden of genetic disease we have, at Chalk River, over the past fifteen years or so, been engaged in integrating into individual and family histories, the vital and health records for British Columbia. Computers are used to link birth registrations back to the parental marriage registrations, and to link records of deaths, registerable handicaps, hospital discharges, and those of a government surveillance scheme for congenital malformations, back to the birth records of the individuals concerned. The resulting individual and kinship histories now include information relating to some 1.5 million vital and health "events" in the lives of well over a half million persons born from 1946 onward. Computer methods have had to be developed to handle all of the work; we simply could not afford to do it all clerically.

The integrated magnetic tape files have been used in a variety of ways, e.g. to: a) obtain data on the numbers of persons suffering from various hereditary and partially hereditary diseases; b) study the strengths of the familiar associations of various diseases; c) look for possible effects of a supposed accumulation of naturally occurring mutations in aging parents, as evidence for a mutational component in disease; and d) detect possible differentials of fertility which might selectively maintain in the population the frequencies of the causal genes.

Such work is very different from, for example, that of carrying out a host mediated assay to test an environmental chemical for mutagenic activity. This difference serves to emphasize the need to consider seriously just where the priorities of geneticists in such matters ought to lie. Concern over the effects of mutations on human health has in the past come mainly from those geneticists who are occupied with studying tthe production of mutations in the laboratory, in lower organisms. Here an anomaly exists which needs to be pointed out.

It is a matter of conviction in such circles that any increase in the mutation rate in man will have important effects on his future health and well-being. This may or may not be true. And yet few geneticists appear especially concerned with establishing this simple belief, in quantitative form, on a scientific basis. But this is precisely what needs to be done, and it would be difficult indeed to do it without adequate data on human disease. Thus a shift in emphasis on the part of geneticists would seem unavoidable if they wish to be convincing in their concern over the impact of mutations on human health, and if they wish to advise society in a realistic fashion for its own protection. I would suggest that the highest priority should be given to this transition.

If the problem of man-made mutagens is as important to society as many geneticists feel it to be, they should no longer be satisfied with piecemeal approaches to the strictly relevant unsolved problems of human population genetics. Fortunately, it is now becoming increasingly possible to tap the vast quantities of information on family relationships, fertility, mortality, and disease that are recorded routinely for individuals throughout whole human populations in developed countries.

GENETIC EXPERIMENTS ON HEALTH AND FITNESS OF EXPERIMENTAL MAMMALIAN POPULATIONS

THOMAS H. RODERICK

The primary concern of this conference has been the available methods and potential methods for detecting increased mutation rates in human populations. Also receiving considerable attention from the participants was the question of ultimate consequence to human health of a specific increase in the mutation rate. Dr. Howard B. Newcombe has repeatedly emphasized that this second question is the one of major concern and is an area of some of our greatest scientific ignorance (see these Proceedings, and for example Newcombe, 1975). It was fitting and valuable for the participants to ponder these two questions together during the course of this conference.

This second question concerns the so-called "mixed bag" of human diseases, which have at least a genetic component in their etiology but for which the inheritance is complicated, which may occur respectively anytime during life from birth to old age, which have a great range of debilitating effects from severe to imperceptible, and which, as a group of diseases of those at least in part of genetic origin, probably produce the greatest health and economic burden to humanity. So, although we are on comparatively firm ground in estimating the consequences of increased mutation rates to the incidences of diseases of simple dominant, recessive, or X-linked inheritance and even those due to well-defined chromosomal aberrations, we know almost nothing of the change of incidence of these other diseases of more complex genitic etiology.

Even during the early 1950's when Dr. W. L. Russell was working with considerable success on estimating risks from irradiation using specific loci in mice, other scientists were using mice with less success in an attempt to determine the heritable effects of irradiation on general health and fitness. Several recent reviews e.g. Green 1968, Newcombe 1971, UNSCEAR 1972) cover the literature well, but it is worth noting that many investigators ultimately became actively concerned. These included Charles, Carter, Green, Newcombe, Lüning, Gowen, Touchberry, Chapman, Spalding, Cox, Godfrey, King, Searle,

Ehling, Sugahara, Sheridan, Russell, Grahn, Havenstein, Verley, Taylor, Soares, and many others. Most of this work in mammals was done in mice or rats, the treatment was usually X-irradiation, the exposures were sometimes given to several consecutive generations with doses as high as 900R to sperm or spermatogonia, and with many various endpoints of concern including life-time reproductive performance, number born, mortality in utero, mortality between birth and weaning, number exhibiting phenotypic deviations, life span, radiation restistance, spontaneous activity, body weight, sex-ratio, maze performance, and several others. These were empirical studies really designed to "see what happens". Although considerable useful information came from this work I think it is fair to say that we still have relatively little idea of the decrement in health and fitness from more than one generation of irradiation to mammals. In an early conference on this subject (Roderick 1964) this lack of a clearly detectable heritable effect led one participant to proffer a "Hurrah" because the effects were perhaps less than anticipated. But it led others to wonder if we were measuring the most sensitive endpoints. Others were further concerned that rodents because they are polytocous are not good models for understanding effects in monotocous man because lowered fitness leading to loss of a rodent embryo might be compensated, masked, confounded, or at least undetected.

But regardless of these experimental problems, on can say from the long-term multi-generation experiments of E. L. Green (several generations of 900R to spermatogonia), K. G. Lüning (several generations of 276R to spermatogonia), and J. F. Spalding, the consequences to the fitness of mouse populations maintained in the laboratory were for the most part undetectable and therefore negligible. Spalding's experiment is the only one still continuing, now having passed its 70th consecutive generation of 200R of spermatogonial X-irradiation (Spalding 1975). The others were either terminated with relief by the investigators or by necessity because of dwindling federal interest and support for such projects in the United States.

There are two further issues which have an important bearing on the problem of genetic fitness of individuals and populations. One is the question of the extent of the dominant effects on fitness of recessive lethals or recessive detrimentals in mammals. Are these effects negligible? The other is the extent to which mammals may be similar to drosophila in having a greatly increased number of mutations with minor deleterious effects relative to the number of mutations with major lethal or near-lethal effects (Mukai 1964, discussed in BEIR 1972). If mice are similar, and if these loci are as mutable as commonly studied mammalian loci, then the consequences to health would be severe for an increased mutation rate. Both these issues need study, and the answers will not come easiliy or quickly.

Our ignorance in this area for mammals is not much advanced beyond that of 10 to 20 years ago. We should ask ourselves whether our methodologies or approaches in mammalian genetics have advanced sufficiently in recent years to make it feasible or worthwhile to attack this problem again experimentally. Are we ready again for long-term experiments in mammalian mutation research? Or are there other ways to get the information?

REFERENCES

BEIR: The Effects on Populations of exposure to low levels of ionizing radiation. Report of the Advisory Committee on the Biological Effects of Ionizing Radiations (so-called Beir Committee), National Academy of Sciences, National Research Council, Washington, D.C. (1972)

Green, E. L.: Genetic effect of radiation on mammalian populations. Annual Rev. of Genetics 2, 87–120 (1968)

Mukai, T.: The genetic structure of natural populations: I. Spontaneous mutation rate of polygenes controlling viability. Genetics 40, 1–19 (1964)

Newcombe, H. B.: The genetic effets of ionizing radiations. Adv. in Genetics 16, 239–303. Academic Press, New York (1971)

Newcombe, H. B.: Mutation and the amount of human ill health. Part of a symposium on New Ways of Estimating Genetic Risks in Man. Proceedings of the 5th International Congress of Radiation Research, Seattle, Washington, July 1974 (1975)

Roderick, T. H. (ed.): Proceedings of the Symposium: The Effects of Radiation on the Hereditary Fitness of Mammalian Populations. Genetics 50, 1023–1217 (1964)

Spalding, J. F.: Some observations on the comparative effects of inbreeding and whole-body X-ray exposure to seventy generations of mice. Los Alamos Scientific Laboratory informal report No. LA-5866-MS (1975)

UNSCEAR: Ionizing Radiation: Levels and Effects. A report of the United Nations Scientific Committee on the Effects of Atomic Radiation to the General Assembly. Volumes I and II. United Nations Publication Sales Numbers E.72.IX.17, and E.72.IX.18, United Nations, New York (1972)

ARE CYTOGENETIC STUDIES ON LYMPHOCYTE CULTURES OF EXPOSED PERSONS A VALID MUTAGENICITY TEST? DATA ON 67 PATIENTS TREATED WITH CYTOSTATIC DRUGS

A. SCHINZEL AND W. SCHMID

Lymphocyte cultures from persons exposed to possibly mutagenic substances are sometimes considered to be an especially relevant test for mutagenicity. The purpose of the present investigation was to submit to a test the reliability of that opinion. Chromosome preparations were made from 73 lymphocyte cultures from 67 patients under cytostatic or immunosuppressive therapy and from 10 healthy control persons. The therapeutically used drugs included alkylating agents (Cyclophosphamide, Busulfan, Chlorambucil, Nitrogen Mustard, L-Phenylalanine Mustard, Procarbazine, BCNU and CCNU), antibiotics (Actionomycin D, Adriamycin, Bleomycin and Daupomycin), antimetabolites (Methotrexate, 6-Mercaptopurine, Azathioprine, Thioguanine, Cytosine Arabinoside, 5-Fluorouracil, Hydroxyurea and L-Asparaginase) and mitotic spindle inhibitors (Vincristine Sulfat and Vinblastine). In addition, some patients had therapeutic irradiation. Almost every patient had received combined therapy with several drugs. If possible, 100 metaphases were scored for structural aberrations of chromatid type (gaps, breaks and exchanges) and chromosome type (rings, dicentrics, acentric fragments, and abnormal chromosomes). The incidence of mitoses with *chromatid breaks and exchanges* in 77 cases ranged from 0 to 4 % in patients and controls, and was independent of the presence of chromosome type aberrations; furthermore, it did not appear to correlate to the type and dose of the drugs received. The same lack of correlation applies to 6 persons in whose cultures 5–15 % of the mitoses contained chromosome breaks and exchanges. The incidence of mitoses with *chromosome type aberrations* did not exceed 1 % in all controls nor in 19 out of 20 patients who had received antimetabolites and spindle inhibitors only. Out of 53 patients who had received alkylating agents, cytostatic antibiotics or X-rays, the incidence of mitoses with chromosome type aberrations was 0–1 % in 22 and 2–29 % in 31 persons. Presence and incidence of chromosome type aberrations did not correlate with the doses of cytostatic drugs they had received. Except for the 6 patients under Bleomycin-treatment, patients were found for each agent tested exhibiting no more than 1 % of mitoses with chromosome type aberrations. The results of these examinations, i.e. no increase of chromatid breaks and exchanges and an inconstant increase of chromosome type aberrations in lymphocyte chromosomes from patients who had received high doses of agents with known chromosome breaking activity implicate that cytogenetic examinations on lymphocyte cultures of exposed persons cannot be considered a valid screening test for weak or questionable mutagens. It is better to direct the efforts to *in vivo* bone marrow tests combined with *in vitro* tests on cultured cells.

THE FATE OF NEW MUTATIONS IN EXPERIMENTAL POPULATIONS OF DROSOPHILA

D. SPERLICH

Monitoring human populations for increased mutation rates is a very important task indeed. Without knowing the further fate of induced mutations, however, no final conclusions can be drawn. Studies on experimental populations of Drosophila may provide, however, some general information about the effect of newly induced mutations on the population level.

Observing experimental populations of D.melanogaster we found that the classical assume of independently selected genes is certainly not correct. The fate of mutations depends evidently not only on their own specific effects on fitness but also on the genetic background in which they happen to arise and on the group of genes with which they happen to come into linkage.

Populations of D.melanogaster made homozygous for their second chromosomes incorporated in almost all cases introduced lethal chromosomes with the dominant markers L and Cy into their gene pools by establishing balanced systems. In genetically heterogeneous populations, however, introduced LCy-chromosomes disappeared very soon from the gene pool. Very similar results could be observed when the fate of X-ray induced recessive lethals was followed. In homozygous populations some of the lethals were heterotic and, therefore, reached a comparably high frequency, whereas in heterogeneous populations no balanced, X-ray induced lethals could be found. Starting with lethal free populations, the frequency increase of spontaneous lethals was higher in homozygous than in heterozygous populations with a high level of genetic variability. Again, some of the spontaneous lethals proved heterotic in one or the other homozygous but never in a heterozygous population. EMS induced lethals, however, can be heterotic in homo- and heterozygous populations as well.

In a set of other experimental populations of D.melanogaster the effect of linkage was studied. As a model, populations were constructed containing the recessive markers dp and b on one and the $+^{dp}+^{b}$ alleles on the other second chromosomes. The populations were started with heterozygous dpb/++ individuals. One group of populations had only little genetic variability in so far as all dpb and all + + chromosomes were isogenic. This group of populations many be called monochromosomal populations. The other group contained many different dpb and + + chromosomes and the populations were called polychromosomal populations. The markers dp and b can be mapped on the second chromosome apart from each other with a distance of 35.5 linkage units. Since the populations were started with chromosomes in coupling phase only, they were at the beginning in a complete linkage disequlibirium. As expected, the repulsion chromosomes dp + and +b were then produced by crossing over every generation and the populations approached linkage equilibrium with generations elapsed. Monochromosomal populations, however, reached their equilibria in all cases less rapidly than polychromosomal populations. The difference may be due to gene interaction favoring the coupling phase chromosomes or to a hitch-hiking effect which is more effective in the monochromosomal populations in which the b locus was heterotic. Whatever the case may be, however, the fate of the markers depends on linkage. A small experiment with X-ray induced lethals on the dpb chromosome showed that the same phenomenon can be observed for new mutations. It is clear from these experiments that linkage and maybe interaction play an important role in the determination of the fate of induced mutations.

DIFFERENCES IN PATERNAL AGE AND THEIR POSSIBLE IMPACT ON MUTATION RATES

WILHELM TÜNTE

As early as in 1912 Weinberg has noted a positive birth order effect in sporadic cases with achondroplasia which, in his view, might suggest mutational origin. Not until some 45 years later Penrose has shown that the association with birth order is in fact due to advanced paternal age. Since then numerous publications have dealt with the age-dependency of spontaneous mutations not only for achondroplasia, but also for acrocephalosyndactyly, myositis ossificans progressiva and Marfan syndrome.

There are two different approaches for studying the association between mutation and paternal age. The first one which has commonly been used hitherto, is characterized by starting from individuals carrying a dominant mutant gene and subsequent searching for the age of the father at the patient's birth. This approach aims at the question whether a presumptive correlation between the incidence of a specific mutation and the age of the father can or cannot be demonstrated. The second approach presupposes some age-dependent mutations and investigates the question to what extent mutation rates in distinct populations might differ because of different paternal age distributions. The following paper is based on the latter approach. It aims at 3 questions:

1. How wide is the range of variation in paternal age as observed in present human populations? In which populations do we find the highest and in which the lowest proportion of older fathers and how much might they consequently differ on this behalf in their mutation rates?
2. What paternal age differences do exist, say, between the turn of the last century and the present time? Considering the well-known secular decrease in paternal age, how much might it have reduced the mutation rates?
3. Is there any evidence for different paternal age distributions in different occupational groups? What might be the consequences in respect to mutations rates?

Since the exact reference population is not known and since paternal age data are rather scanty in most mutation studies, we have calculated relative incidence figures according to the following method:
If p_x means the proportion of patients' fathers, belonging to age group x, and if q_x indicates the corresponding proportion of fathers in the total population, then the "relative risk" would be $R_x = \frac{p_x}{q_x}$. The age-specific risk figures are multiplied with the appropriate proportions of the population under study. The sum of all these products is then denoted as the "relative incidence". Such incidence figures calculated

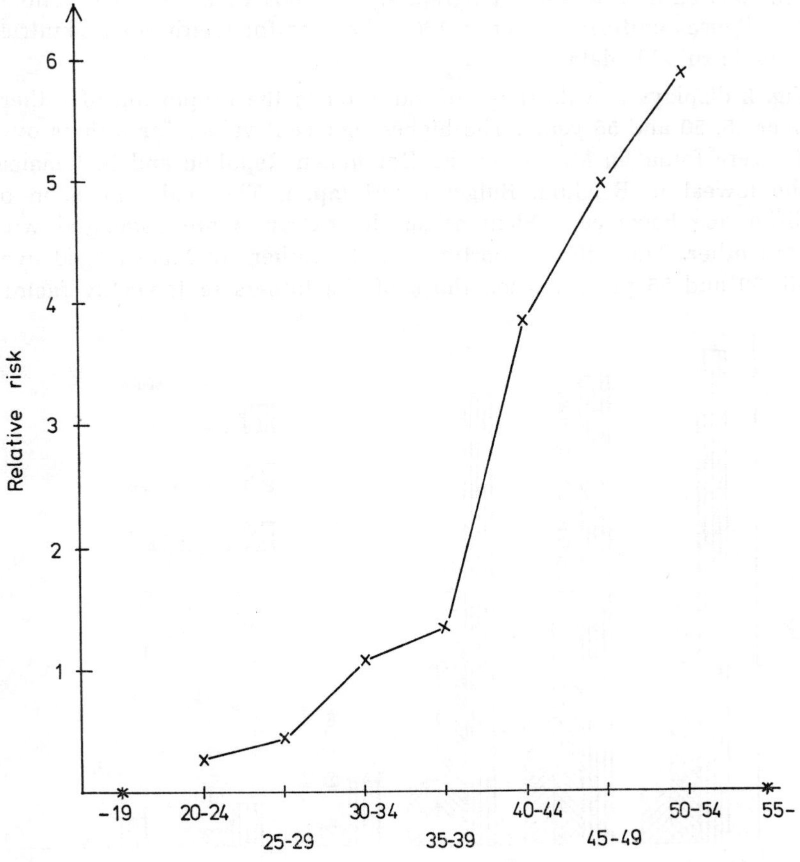

Fig. 1: Paternal age in mutations for achondroplasia (after Murdoch et al. 1970)

for different paternal age distributions may easily be compared with each other since the actual numbers of fathers do not enter the formula. The following calculations are restricted to mutations for achondroplasia which show a clear paternal age effect. They are based on the age-specific relative risk figures given by Murdoch et al. and presented in the graph on page 135 (Fig. 1).

1. Differences between present populations

In order to study the influence of different paternal age distributions found in present populations, the relevant data were extracted from the 1969 edition of the Demographic Yearbook of the United Nations. The figures uniformly refer to 1963, the year for which most countries provide suitable data.

Fig. 2 displays a wide range of variation in the proportion of fathers over 45, 50 and 55 years. The highest per cent values for fathers over 45 were found in Macau, in the Dominican Republic and in Jamaica, the lowest in Belgium, Bulgaria and Japan. The real dimension of difference becomes evident when the extremes are compared with each other. Thus, the proportions of the fathers in Macau aged over 45, 50 and 55 years exceed those of the fathers in Japan by factors

Fig. 2: Paternal age in different countries (legitimate live births 1963)

of 16.7, 15.6 and 18, respectively. The remaining 40 populations tested range between Jamaica and Belgium whereby the percentage of fathers over 45 is still higher than 10 % in Martinique, Guadeloupe, El Salvador, and Venezuela.

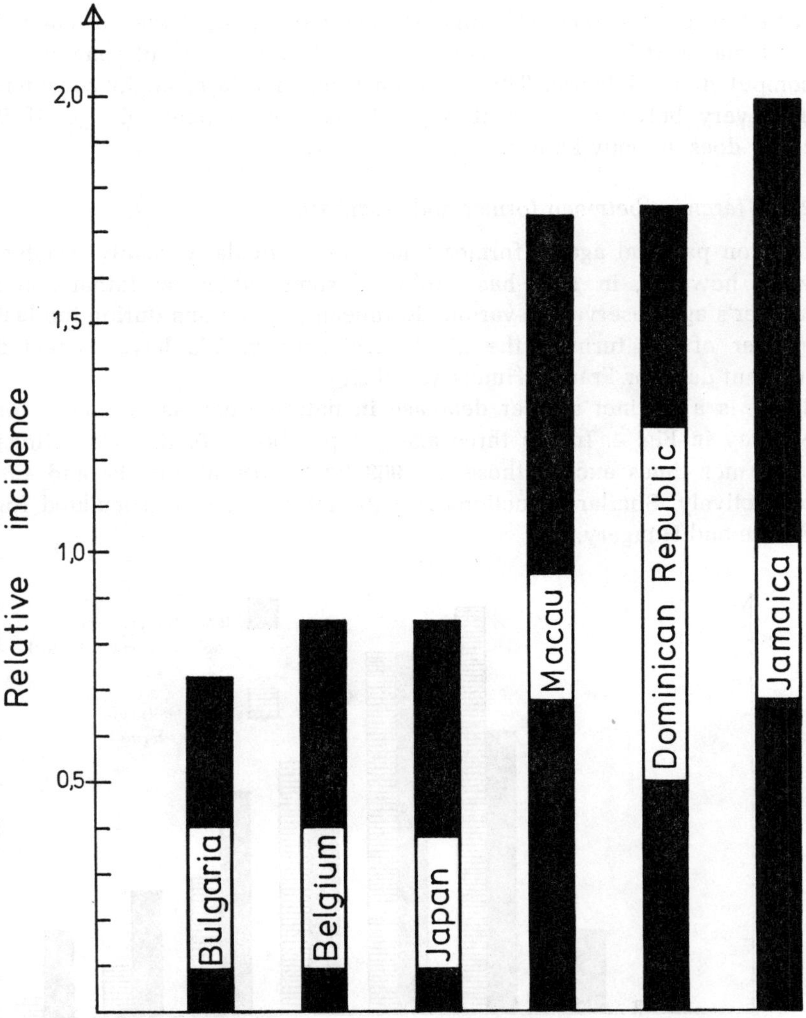

Fig. 3: Relative incidence of mutations for achondroplasia in different countries

If the relative incidence figures are calculated for the six countries with the most extreme age distributions, the above mentioned results are obtained (Fig. 3).

As we would expect there are greatly different incidence figures between the countries with high proportions of older fathers and those with low proportions. The highest figure of about 2 was calculated for Jamaica. It is 2.7 times as high as the lowest figure of roughly 0.7 computed for Bulgaria. The mutation rate, therefore, might considerably vary between different populations due to paternal age. If it really does, nobody knows.

2. *Differences between former and recent times*

Data on paternal age in former times are particularly scanty. Wedervang, however, in 1924 has published some tables on father's and mother's age observed in various European populations during the last quarter of the turn of the nineteenth century. We have extracted relevant data for France, Hungary and Norway.

There is a distinct secular decrease in paternal age as is shown for Norway in Fig. 4. In the three age groups above 40, the proportions of former times exceed those of 1963 by factors of 1.6, 2.4 and 4.6, respectively. Similar reductions in paternal age can be calculated for France and Hungary.

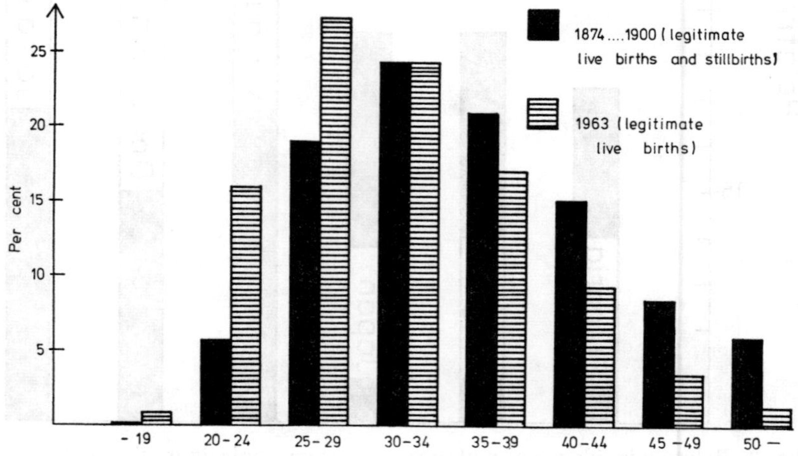

Fig. 4: Paternal age at different times in Norway (in years)

The corresponding relative incidence figures are graphically presented in Fig. 5.

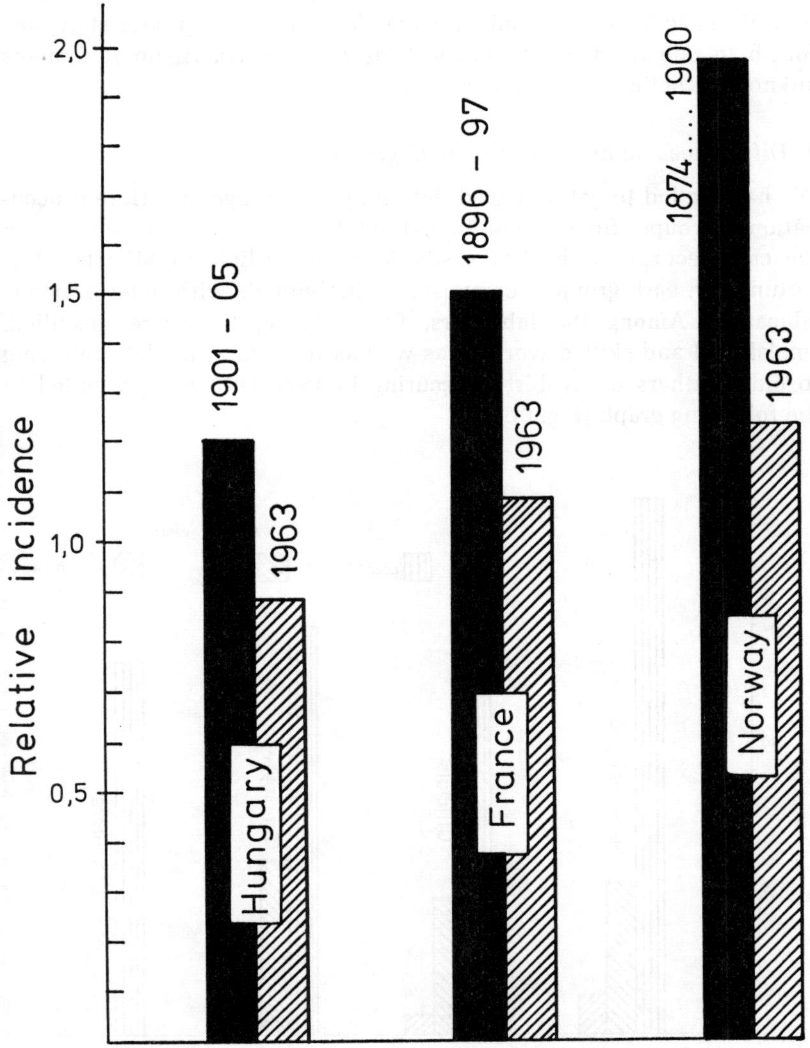

Fig. 5: Relative incidence of mutations for achondroplasia in different countries at different times

As we would assume, a decrease of the relative incidence of mutations for achondroplasia is found for all three populations. It almost amounts to 26.9 % for Hungary, to 27.7 % for France, and to 37.6 % for Norway. This means that due to reduced paternal age the number of mutations for this specific disease might have declined by approximately one fourth to one third during the last 70 years or so. Again it remains unknown whether such a decline has in fact occurred.

3. Differences between professional groups

We have failed to get unbiased data on paternal age in different occupational groups. So we had to extract the corresponding data from the case records of the University Maternity Clinic in Münster. Unfortunately, each group is composed of individuals with heterogeneous education. Among the labourers, for instance, there are unskilled, semiskilled and skilled workers as well as foreman. The data referring to older fathers of livebirths occuring in 1971–1973 are presented in the following graph (Fig. 6).

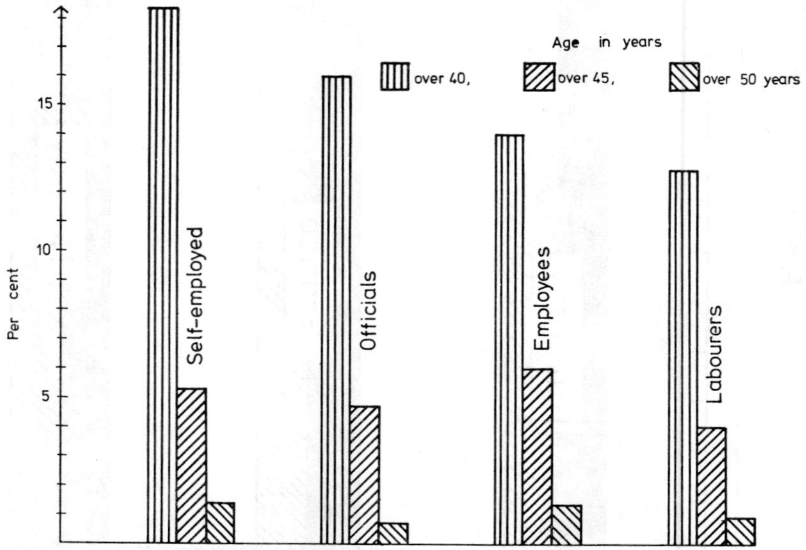

Fig. 6: Paternal age in different professional groups (University Maternity Clinic Münster, 1971–73)

No consistent trend of the proportions of fathers aged above 45 or 50 can be observed when the groups are arranged in the proposed order. There is, however, a slight continuous decline in the proportion of fathers aged above 40, ranging from 18.3 % in the self-employed down to 12.8 % in the labourers. The appropriate relative incidence figures are graphically presented in Fig. 7.

A rather steady, slight increase in the relative incidence can be seen, beginning with about 1.2 in the group of the employees and ending with almost 1.5 in the group of the self-employed. We might then conclude that mutations for achondroplasia may occur slightly more often in the group of the self-employed than in the group of the employees although nothing is actually known on this point.

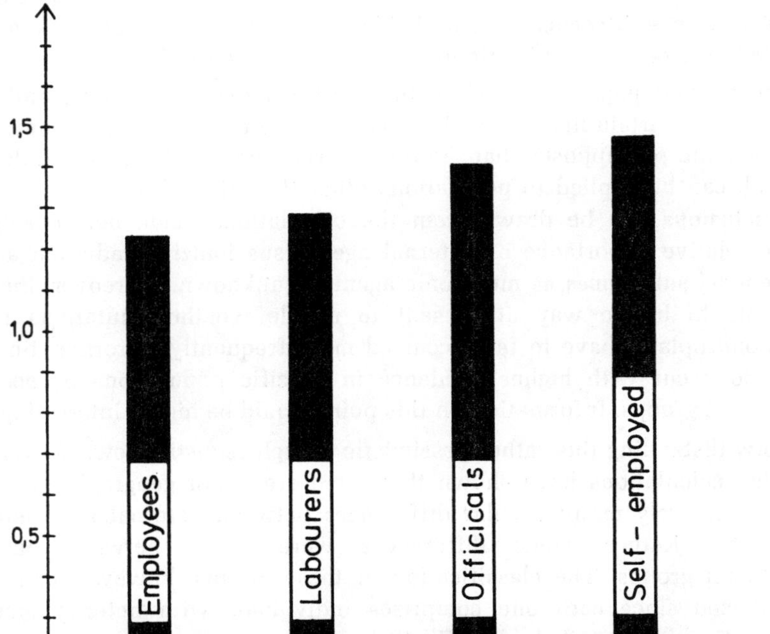

Fig. 7: Relative incidence of mutations for achondroplasia in different professional groups

Concluding remarks

The causes of spontaneous mutations are widely unknown. Paternal age has been proven as a rather clear-cut factor correlated with mutations for four autosomal dominant disorders among which achondroplasia is a well-known example.

Apart from this group, Vogel distinguishes a second group of other dominant mutations, comprising neurofibromatosis, tuberous sclerosis, osteogenesis imperfecta and probably others which seem to be only slightly influenced by paternal age as indicated indirectly by an analysis of the birthorder. Although the evidence for such a slight paternal age effect appears to be rather weak, it cannot be overlooked that sporadic cases with other rare dominant diseases are not infrequently associated with an elevated age of the father (Jones et al., 1975). Hence, it seems quite probable that paternal age plays a greater role in the causation of mutations than we are aware of.

The present paper has dealt with a rather hypothetical topic and is subject to certain limitations. It is restricted to mutations for achondroplasia and presupposes that the relative risk figures given by Murdoch et al. can be applied to populations other than the USA. No practical conclusions can be drawn from the calculations made before since the relative importance of paternal age versus ionizing radiation and chemical substances as mutagenic agents is unknown. Moreover, there seems to be no way at present to decide whether mutations for achondroplasia have in fact occurred more frequently in former times or do occur with higher incidence in specific populations or occupational groups. Information on this point would be highly interesting.

Notwithstanding this rather pessimistic though realistic view, the foregoing calculations have shown that there are major geographical and comparatively minor secular differences between paternal age distributions. Rather vague differences were found between occupational groups. The classification of these groups, however, can be criticized since each one comprises individuals with heterogeneous education. A detailed classification more appropriate to schooling seems desirable.

The differences in paternal age analysed in a fairly large number of populations, suggest a wide variation in the relative incidence of mutations for achondroplasia, varying from approximately 0.7 to about 2, i.e. by a factor of 2.7. Based on secular changes in paternal age since the turn of the last century, the relative incidence figures calculated for some European populations could be shown to range at most from around 1.2 to almost 2 or, in other words, by a factor of 1.6. The relative figures differed only little between the occupational groups. The findings show that the observed differences in paternal age might induce a wide variation in the rate of mutations for achondroplasia, an effect which of course may be masked by a great variety of other mutagenic influences.

REFERENCES

Jones, K.L., D.W. Smith, M.A. Sedgwick Harvey, B.D. Hall, and L. Quan: Older paternal age and fresh gene mutation: data on additional disorders. J. Pediatr. 86, 84–88 (1975)

Murdoch, J.L., B.A. Walker, J.G. Hall, H. Abbey, K.K. Smith, and V.A. McKusick: Achondroplasia – a genetic and statistical survey. Ann.Hum.Genet. (Lond.) 33, 227 (1970)

Penrose, L.S.: Parental age and mutation. Lancet II, 312 (1955)

Vogel, F.: Spontaneous mutation in man. In: Chemical mutagenesis in mammals and man. Ed. by Vogel, F., and G. Röhrborn. Springer, Berlin, Heidelberg, New York 1970 (p. 16)

Wedervang, I.: Om seksualproporsjonen ved fødselen. Steenske Forlag, Oslo 1924

Weinberg, W.: Zur Vererbung des Zwergwuchses. Arch.Rassenbiol. 9, 710 (1912)

LIST OF PARTICIPANTS

Dr. S. Abrahamson	Department of Zoology The University of Wisconsin Madison, Wisconsin 53706/USA
Dr. E. Albert	Kinderklinik der Universität München Pettenkoferstr. 8a 8000 München
Dr. K. Altland	Institut für Anthropologie und Humangenetik der Universität Heidelberg Im Neuenheimer Feld 328 6900 Heidelberg
Dr. A. Basler	Institut für Humangenetik und Anthropologie der Universität Düsseldorf Ulenbergstr. 127–129 4000 Düsseldorf
Dr. J. A. Beardmore	University College of Swansea Department of Genetics Singleton Park Swansea SA2 8PP/UK
Dr. H. Beikirch	Zentrallaboratorium für Mutagenitätsprüfung Breisacherstr. 33 7800 Freiburg/Breisgau
Dr. K. Bender	Institut für Humangenetik und Anthropologie der Universität Freiburg Albertstr. 11 7800 Freiburg/Breisgau
Dr. G. Beyaert	Zentrallaboratorium für Mutagenitätsprüfung Breisacherstr. 33 7800 Freiburg/Breisgau

Dr. A. Bodenberger	Zentrallaboratorium für Mutagenitätsprüfung Breisacherstr. 33 7800 Freiburg/Breisgau
Dr. C. Bresch	Institut für Biologie III der Universität Freiburg Schänzlestr. 9–11 7800 Freiburg/Breisgau
Dr. J. F. Crow	The University of Wisconsin Genetics Building Madison, Wisconsin 53706/USA
Dr. K.-H. Degenhardt	Institut für Humangenetik der Universität Frankfurt Paul-Ehrlich-Str. 41 6000 Frankfurt
P. Dinger	Zentrallaboratorium für Mutagenitätsprüfung Breisacherstr. 33 7800 Freiburg/Breisgau
J. Ellenberger	Zentrallaboratorium für Mutagenitätsprüfung Breisacherstr. 33 7800 Freiburg/Breisgau
Dr. W. Engel	Institut für Humangenetik und Anthropologie der Universität Freiburg Albertstr. 11 7800 Freiburg/Breisgau
Dr. H. J. Evans	MRC Clinical and Population Cytogenetics Unit Western General Hospital Edinburgh EH4 2XU/UK
Dr. R. Fahrig	Zentrallaboratorium für Mutagenitätsprüfung Breisacherstr. 33 7800 Freiburg/Breisgau
Dr. H. Galjaard	Erasmus Universiteit Rotterdam Faculty of Medicine Dept. Cell Biology & Genetics Postbus 1738 Rotterdam/The Netherlands

Dr. E. Günther | Max-Planck-Institut für Immunbiologie
Stübeweg 51
7800 Freiburg/Breisgau

Dr. R. L. Hausmann | Institut für Biologie III der Universität Freiburg
Schänzlestr. 9–11
7800 Freiburg/Breisgau

Dr. S. Hollan | National Institute of Haematology and Blood Transfusion
Daróczi ut 24
1113 Budapest/Hungary

Dr. J. Klose | Pharmakologisches Institut d. Freien Universität Berlin
Embryonal-Pharmakologie
Thielallee 69/73
1000 Berlin 33

Dr. C. H. Langley | Population Genetics and Epidemiology
Environmental Mutagenesis Branch
N.I.E.H.S.
P.O. Box 12233
Research Triangle Park, N.C. 27709/USA

Dr. A. Lengeróva | Institute of Experimental Biology and Genetics
Czechoslovak Academy of Sciences
Prague/CSSR

Dr. A. Leonard | Centre d'Etude de l'Energie Nucléaire
Laboratoires du C.E.N./S.C.K.
Mol/Belgium

Dr. J. Neel | The University of Michigan
Dept. of Human Genetics
Ann Arbor, Michigan 48104/USA

Dr. V. Neuhoff | Max-Planck-Institut für Exp. Medizin
Forschungsstelle Neurochemie
Hermann-Rein-Str. 3
3400 Göttingen

Dr. H. Newcombe | Atomic Energy of Canada Ltd.
Biology and Health Physics Division
Chalk River, Ontario KOJ 1JO/CDN

T. H. Roderick	Energy Research and Development Administration Division of Biomedical and Environmental Research Washington, D.C. 20545/USA
Dr. A. Schinzel	Universitäts-Kinderklinik Genetisches Labor Steinwiesstr. 75 Zürich/Switzerland
Dr. W. Schmid	Universitäts-Kinderklinik Genetisches Labor Steinwiesstr. 75 Zürich/Switzerland
Dr. L. Schoeller	Zentrallaboratorium für Mutagenitätsprüfung Breisacherstr. 33 7800 Freiburg/Breisgau
Dr. D. Sperlich	Institut für Biologie II der Universität Tübingen Abt. Populationsgenetik Auf der Morgenstelle 28 7400 Tübingen
Dr. W. Tünte	Institut für Humangenetik der Universität Münster Vesaliusweg 12/14 4400 Münster/Westf.
Dr. F. Vogel	Institut für Anthropologie und Humangenetik der Universität Heidelberg Im Neuenheimer Feld 328 6900 Heidelberg
Dr. D. Wild	Zentrallaboratorium für Mutagenitätsprüfung Breisacherstr. 33 7800 Freiburg/Breisgau
Dr. U. Wolf	Institut für Humangenetik und Anthropologie der Universität Freiburg Albertstr. 11 7800 Freiburg/Breisgau